HOME care AND HOSPICE

STAFF COMPETENCE

EXAMPLES OF COMPLIANCE

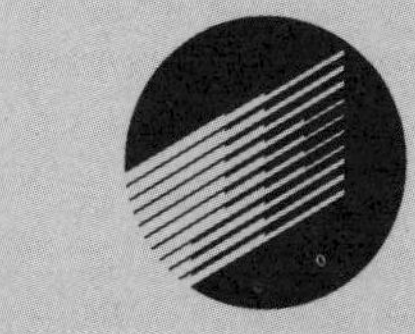

Joint Commission

Joint Commission Mission

The mission of the Joint Commission on Accreditation of Healthcare Organizations is to improve the quality of care provided to the public through the provision of health care accreditation and related services that support performance improvement in health care organizations.

Joint Commission educational programs and publications support, but are separate from, the accreditation activities of the Joint Commission. Attendees at Joint Commission educational programs and purchasers of Joint Commission publications receive no special consideration or treatment in, or confidential information about, the accreditation process.

An exhaustive effort has been made to locate all persons having any rights or interests in material and to clear reprint permissions. If any required acknowledgments have been omitted or any rights overlooked, it is unintentional.

Printed in the U.S.A. 5 4 3 2 1

Requests for permission to reprint or make copies of any part of this book should be mailed to:
Permissions Editor
Department of Publications
Joint Commission on Accreditation of Healthcare Organizations
One Renaissance Boulevard
Oakbrook Terrace, IL 60181

ISBN: 0-86688-555-2

Library of Congress Catalog Card Number: 97-74777

For more information about the Joint Commission,
please contact our Web site at http://www.jcaho.org

CONTENTS

Introduction

The demands on health care professionals and organizations seem to expand daily, and chief among these demands is the need for high-quality care delivered in the most cost-effective manner and setting possible. Home care and hospice organizations have helped meet this need by providing care and services to a growing mix of patients with increasingly complex care needs. Managed care organizations, third-party payers, accrediting bodies, and consumers are relying on home care and hospice providers more than ever before and are evaluating these providers with much the same attention previously reserved for acute care settings.

In this environment, employees are the most important resource an organization has, and their ability to deliver care and services appropriately and efficiently is crucial to that organization's survival. Staff members' abilities, or competencies, are often the greatest determinant of the quality of care provided. Thus, organizations need to make the optimization of staff capabilities a top priority. They need to establish programs to assess their employees' skills, identify education and training needs, and help them maintain and improve their proficiencies.

The Joint Commission's management of human resources standards from the *Comprehensive Accreditation Manual for Home Care* identify the components of an effective competence assessment process and provide a framework for developing a systematic, organizationwide program. Because competency standards were only introduced to the home care field with the 1995 edition of the manual, they are still relatively new to many organizations and some confusion still exists about how to use them to the best advantage.

The purpose of this book is to help home care and hospice organizations understand the key issues and challenges involved with ensuring that home care organizations have competent staff. It identifies relevant Joint Commission standards as well as common problems the field may encounter during implementation and describes the basic components of the survey process that pertain to competence assessment.

The book is divided into three chapters. Chapter 1 provides key background information on the importance of patient care staff competency to all home care and hospice organizations. It also explains Joint Commission requirements for competency.

Chapter 2 addresses the survey process. It describes the survey activities in which organizations are expected to demonstrate compliance with the competency standards and explains the relationship between performance improvement and a competence assessment program.

Chapter 3 is the core of the book. It provides numerous real-world examples of how all types of home care and hospice organizations have demonstrated compliance with Joint Commission competency standards. These examples, which have been reviewed and in many cases recommended by Joint Commission surveyors, are intended to serve as models for adaptation by individual organizations and to encourage creativity and innovation in meeting competence assessment requirements. However, it is important to note that the activities, processes, forms, and so on presented in the examples are not required by the Joint Commission standards.

The examples are separated into three sections:

- **Planning for competent staff.** These examples include organizations' development plans, inventories of competencies, and other tools and procedures used to establish a competence assessment program.

- **Assessing individual competence.** This section presents example assessment tools from a wide variety of organizations, covering many different types of positions.

- **Maintaining and improving staff competence.** This section includes tools for gathering data related to staff competency, staff education materials, and policies and procedures for ongoing evaluation of proficiency.

In addition, an appendix offers a checklist staff can use to assess their compliance with Joint Commission standards.

Home Care and Hospice Staff Competence: Examples of Compliance is designed to help organization leaders, managers, and staff understand the challenges of, and need for, an effective competence assessment program. Furthermore, it shows how organizations can take advantage of the framework provided by Joint Commission standards to achieve such a program.

CHAPTER 1

An important aspect of home care or hospice services—and one of the reasons competence assessment is so important in this field—is that there is no ready access to other professionals when problems arise. Unlike health care professionals in an acute care setting, home care staff are usually alone when delivering care and services, and support—especially across large rural areas—is often unobtainable. In order to handle both routine procedures and emergency situations, their skills and knowledge must be kept current.

As patient populations for home care become more diversified, the competencies required for individual caregivers may change from year to year. For example, the increase in the number of elderly patients, especially the frail elderly, requires many home health nurses to be proficient in specific aspects of geriatric care. As more medically complex patients are discharged "quicker and sicker" from acute care settings, pharmacists will be required to review and demonstrate knowledge of drug interactions prevalent among the types of patients served.

Competence assessment ensures that employees are capable of delivering care or services effectively and efficiently. A number of steps are required to build an organizationwide competence assessment program:

1. Planning to ensure staff competence;

2. Assessing the competence of individual staff members; and

3. Maintaining and improving staff competence on an individual and a collective basis.

These steps are included in the Joint Commission's management of human resources function and reflect several of the basic requirements for standards compliance in this area. Table 1-1 lists the standards from the *Comprehensive Accreditation Manual for Home Care* that apply to competence assessment.

Table 1-1. **Joint Commission Standards Pertaining to Competence Assessment***

HR.1	The leaders provide programs for recruitment, retention, development, and continuing education of all staff members.
HR.2	The organization's leaders define the qualifications for all staff positions.
HR.3.1	The number, qualifications, and health status of staff are appropriate to the scope of care and services provided by the organization.
HR.3.2	The number and qualifications of individuals supervising care and service staff are appropriate to the scope of care and services provided by the organization.
HR.5	The organization has established methods and practices that encourage self-development and learning for all staff.
HR.5.1	The organization provides ongoing education, including in-services, training, and other activities, to maintain and improve staff competence.
HR.6	The organization assesses, maintains, and improves the competence of all care and service staff members.
HR.6.1	The organization collects, aggregates, and analyzes data on staff competence to identify and respond to staff learning needs.

*All of the standards listed apply to competence assessment, although some also include requirements for other aspects of the human resources function.

Source: Joint Commission on Accreditation of Healthcare Organizations: *1997–98 Comprehensive Accreditation Manual for Home Care*. Oakbrook Terrace, IL: Joint Commission, 1996, pp 380–402.

Important Terms

Some organizations use the terms *competence*, *competency*, and *proficiency* to mean different things. Throughout this book, as in the Joint Commission standards, these terms are used interchangeably to mean both the documentation of qualifications (for example, applicable licenses and certification, lists of home care experience) *and* the demonstration of those qualifications in delivering care. In other words, a staff member is able to perform in practice what he or she is qualified to do on paper. *Competence* itself is defined as the possession of the knowledge, skills, and behaviors to perform assigned tasks.

The term *competent staff* includes all full- and part-time employees, contract staff, and volunteers who are involved in patient care, whether directly or indirectly. Based on their organization's mission and scope of care or services, leaders need to define the number of staff necessary to provide care, what the qualifications for each position will be, and what competencies are needed to meet these qualifications.

Staffing and *qualifications*, while related to competence, are separate human resources issues and thus are not covered in detail here. They affect the competence assessment process in the following ways:

- **Number of staff.** Small organizations may have a limited number of employees, requiring existing staff members to take on responsibilities that might not be required of those with similar job descriptions in other facilities. For example, in a large home health agency, a nursing supervisor might not be needed to make home visits and provide hands-on care to patients, unlike a supervisor in a small branch office with limited nursing staff.

- **Staff qualifications.** Qualifications are determined by a variety of elements—law and regulation, individual organizational requirements, needs of the patients being served, and so on. These qualifications are contained in the job description, which in turn is used to identify competencies.

Planning for Competent Staff

The main components of the assessment program that need to be established at the planning stage are as follows:

- What competencies need to be assessed;

- When they should be assessed;

- How they should be assessed and by whom; and

- How they can be improved (that is, what resources will be needed for education and training).

Identifying Competencies

Leaders need to establish what competencies will be required for each employee providing patient care. Job descriptions, which list qualifications and job responsibilities, are a good place to begin. For example, the job description for a respiratory therapist may list responsibilities for setting up a variety of equipment, instructing the patient/family in its use, following up on how the equipment is functioning, and assessing the patient's response to the equipment. Depending on the patients being served, resulting competencies might include apnea monitor set-up, enteral pump set-up, initial assessment of patients receiving oxygen, and documentation.

Competencies can also be identified from studies and research findings conducted within specific fields. For example, in one national study, approximately 360 home health nurse managers listed the knowledge and skills possessed by productive nurses. Thirty-five areas of abilities and knowledge were identified and grouped into like categories to reflect critical job categories. These included practice management, communication, nursing process, home health knowledge, communication, patient/family management, knowledge/skill maintenance, and written documentation.[1]

Projects such as this can provide background information and suggest areas for competence assessment that might not have been evident before. For example, there is often a tendency to focus on clinical and technical aspects of the job when identifying competencies; yet areas such as documentation and communication skills are important as well. The assessment program should cover general competencies that would be necessary to all patient care staff* (for instance, knowledge of safety management) and those that are specific to the employee's job (such as bathing technique) and the organization itself (such as operation of the on-call system). Table 1-2 lists some basic and job-specific competencies for home care.

Another often overlooked area is critical thinking—the ability to draw on previous knowledge and experience, relate it to the current situation, and apply it effectively. It is one of the most important skills any caregiver can possess because it is crucial to establishing, maintaining, and improving competence. For example, a hospice bereavement counselor should be able to assess survivors' needs, such as identifying grief patterns correctly in order to address the survivors' specific needs.

Establishing the Frequency of Assessment

Leaders should define how often assessment needs to take place. This may vary depending on the position, the patient population served (high-risk, problem-prone), and law and regulation for different fields.

Staff members' competence should be assessed

- at the time they are hired;

- after they have received orientation; and

- periodically thereafter.

"Periodically" means that the staff member is reassessed according to applicable law and regulation and the organization's own policies and definitions. He or she is also assessed when given new job responsibilities, when the organization institutes new procedures or techniques, and when new equipment or technology is introduced. The minimal acceptable frequency for any staff member to be assessed in some (not necessarily all) competencies is once within the three-year accreditation cycle.

---

*The term *patient care staff* is used throughout this book to refer to all staff members who are engaged in direct or indirect patient care or care-related services.

Table 1-2. Home Care Competencies

Basic Competencies

- Physical assessment of the patient
- Patient/family education
- Basic life support
- Infection control
- Documentation

- Sterile techniques
- Wound care
- Medication administration
- Venipuncture
- Planning patient care

- Vital signs
- Foley catheter insertion
- Medication compounding
- Equipment calibration and cleaning

Advanced Competencies

- *Diagnosis-specific* competencies for mental health, intrapartum and postpartum, and hospice patients

- *Population-specific* competencies for newborn, infant, child, adolescent, and geriatric assessments

- *Infusion therapy-specific* competencies for blood component and derivatives transfusion, epidural catheter management, and related infusions; total parenteral and enteral nutrition; clinical monitoring of medications; and peripherally inserted central catheter and midline catheter insertion

- *Equipment-specific* competencies for infusion pumps, respiratory or ventilator assistance, dialysis, phototherapy, oxygen concentrator, and apnea monitoring

Source: Adapted from Friedman MM: Competence assessment: How to meet the intent of the Joint Commission on Accreditation of Healthcare Organizations' Management of Human Resources standards. *Home Healthc Nurse* 14(10):772, 1996. Reprinted by permission from Lippincott-Raven Publishers, New York.

Methods of Assessment

There are many ways of assessing competence—observation, written tests, and so on. These are discussed in detail in the next section. At the planning stage, however, leaders should distinguish which competencies require observation and which can be assessed by other methods. For example, reviewing inventory logs, orders, and home care records is probably sufficient to assess a pharmacist's documentation skills, but observation would be necessary to assess aseptic technique and compounding procedures.

Resources for Continuous Improvement

In addition to the assessment process itself, leaders should plan for ongoing maintenance and improvement of staff members' skills. This includes orientation, individualized training, in-services, and other forms of staff development, which are discussed later in this chapter.

The competence assessment program needs to be included in the overall organizational plan to ensure that sufficient resources (both financial and personnel) are anticipated and available. For example, special provisions might be needed to orient, train, and assess staff members who only work weekends and/or evenings.

By committing resources to learning and development activities, leaders send a double message: They are committed to providing patients with the best quality of care possible by providing highly competent staff, and they are committed to helping their employees grow and develop as individuals.

Assessing Individual Competence

Traditionally, assessment has been an informal process, often resulting from a performance deficiency or an adverse patient outcome. A supervisor would discuss the problem with the staff member to identify what skills he or she needed to learn or improve.

Today, competence assessment should be more proactive to ensure that staff are truly capable of delivering high-quality care and services before problems arise. The assessment process should begin with the recruitment and hiring of qualified staff members. Hiring practices should be rigorous in verifying the education, training, skills, and experience needed for each position. This not only aids selection of the most skilled individuals, it establishes a baseline by which to measure future assessments.

The process must allow for verification of paper qualifications and practical demonstration of the abilities inherent in those qualifications. For example, a driver who delivers home medical equipment should be checked to make sure he or she has a current, valid driver's license, good driving record, and experience commensurate with the organization's needs. A supervisor or other qualified person needs to verify through observation that his or her qualifications translate into safe driving; proper delivery and set-up techniques; and effective methods of demonstrating use of the equipment for the patient and ensuring the patient knows how to use the equipment.

Existing staff need to be oriented to both the assessment process and the expectations pertaining to their specific competencies. The latter is especially important if a list of necessary skills/competencies was not included in their original job descriptions. Those who will be responsible for assessing competence also require training and orientation to the process and the materials to be used for documentation.

Levels of Competence

Different categories of home care professionals may be divided into specific levels of competence, which should be taken into consideration during the assessment process. For example, the Dreyfus Skill Acquisition Model is sometimes used to classify nursing competency into five levels:

- **Novice**—new graduate nurse with no experience;

- **Advanced beginner**—independent in some aspects of practice;

- **Competent**—able to apply experience and judgment to new patient situations;

- **Proficient**—efficient at nursing practice; and

- **Expert**—has intuitive grasp of patient care situations.[2]

Such classifications can be adapted for any type of staff member. Although it is not essential to establish formal divisions like these, it is necessary to recognize the different levels and approach assessments accordingly. For example, assessments of employees with less experience could include more field observation of care delivery than reassessments of experienced staff.

Assessment Methods

The Joint Commission competency standards do not require any specific method—only that the methods set down by organization leaders are followed and that these methods are appropriate to the skills being assessed. The basic methods of assessment are observation and documentation. Which methods are used often depends on the types of care and services the organization offers, the number and types of staff it employs, and its resources.

For example, leaders may decide that both observation and documentation are necessary to establish the following competencies for a respiratory therapist:

- Adult and/or pediatric assessment (documentation);

- Performance of routine and preventive maintenance of ventilators (observation);

- Performance of tracheostomy changes (observation);

- Collection of data and interpretation of ventilator settings (documentation); and

- Provision of patient education (observation).

Observation. Those competencies requiring observation for verification should be identified during the leaders' planning stage. Observation may consist of a supervisor, a peer, or someone from another job category accompanying caregivers on home visits and observing their performance of various activities. For example, a Medicare-certified home health agency might send a registered nurse out with home health aides once a year to evaluate areas such as bathing technique, observance of universal precautions, and communication with the patient/family.

Not all observation assessments need to be conducted in the home. Some organizations have "lab settings" in which competencies can be observed for a group of employees outside of the patient's environment. For example, home health aides may be observed taking vital signs on each other or performing CPR on a mannequin in the agency headquarters. Warehouse personnel and pharmacy staff are necessarily observed within their work environments.

In addition to ongoing assessment of frequently performed competencies, organizations may assess workers on a patient-specific basis for special procedures. For example, personal care and support staff may often have little or no training in the use of mechanical lifts, although they are sometimes used in the home. An organization may assess the competence of an employee delivering support services concurrently with training him or her on the lift used in a specific patient's home. The session includes orientation and training, then demonstration of the staff member's ability to use the equipment.

Documentation. There are various ways of assessing competence through documentation. Initial verification of licensure, certification, and past experience should be performed for every employee.

Written tests, skills exams, and audiovisual programs can be used for those competencies not requiring observation. For example, knowledge of medication uses and contraindications could be assessed through a written exam covering topics such as what to look for when evaluating respirations and causes for an apnea monitor to sound an alarm. Other types of competencies that could be evaluated through testing include identification of hazardous materials and wastes, emergency procedures, and disease-specific knowledge.

Review of records and logs could establish whether the staff member is proficient at documenting home visits as well as procedures, such as notification of physicians and communication with other home care professionals.

Maintaining and Improving Competence

A competence program is not solely about assessment. It also involves maintaining and improving existing skills. Organizations need to encourage self-development and continued learning for staff members. Orientation, training programs, and in-service should address those areas identified by competence assessment as needing improvement.

Orientation programs, in addition to including a general introduction to organizationwide policies and procedures, can focus on specific areas identified by competence assessment as problematic for individual job classifications. For example, initial assessments of newly hired registered nurses for a home health organization specializing in pediatric diabetic services might indicate that many nurses, although proficient in performance of venipuncture and wound management, lack experience with pediatric patients, affecting their competency level in patient education. This organization could incorporate the necessary training in the educational needs of this patient population into its orientation program for registered nurses.

Ongoing competency-based education ensures that staff maintain proficiency in areas that are specific to their jobs, their organizations, and the patient populations served. For example, suppose five nurses conduct a group assessment of fifty-two home health aides taking vital signs. Fifty of the aides are proficient at taking temperature, pulse, and respiration, but thirty-eight cannot take blood pressure correctly. An in-service could be conducted on a regular basis until follow-up assessments indicate that the aides are capable of performing this task.

Joint Commission standards require the collection, aggregation, and analysis of data to determine staff learning needs. The assessment process itself involves gathering data. As illustrated in the previous example, combining the assessment findings for each group of employees and keeping track of trends in performance will help leaders plan more efficiently for educational programs and resources.

Assessment data can also be trended for a specific individual to identify a baseline of competence and measure improvements. A new employee might be asked to fill out a skills checklist for self-evaluation of competencies. This self-assessment is then confirmed (or corrected) by a supervisor's assessment and used to establish learning needs and goals. Subsequent assessments (which may be recorded in a matrix throughout the length of employment) track the employee's progress and can proactively identify weak areas.

Ongoing education can take a wide variety of forms, including lectures, one-on-one instruction, audiovisual aids, simulations and role-playing, self-instruction modules, and on-site training. Creativity is often needed to design programs that are effective from both an educational and a cost perspective. Because everyone learns differently, it is helpful to identify staff members' preferred or best ways of learning during the orientation process. For example, some people retain more if they read material rather than having it presented orally. Others cannot seem to grasp a technique from watching someone else; they need to perform the task themselves while being guided by an instructor.

Active learning almost always leads to better retention than traditional classroom teaching alone. In view of this, many organizations hold skills days or equipment days, during which employees can learn about new skills or technology and review existing procedures in an informal atmosphere. One health system developed a "Traveling Salvation Show" to review high-risk/low-frequency skills for critical care nurses. Incorporating games, music, and brightly colored posters in a carnival atmosphere, it involved learners in a flexible, hands-on experience that encouraged participation and critical thinking. Multiple learning methods—from case studies to crossword puzzles to video scenarios—were used to address every level of staff competence in a nonthreatening atmosphere. The entire experience is designed to take each nurse only 45 minutes to complete and reached all required staff during a one-day program. The idea can be adapted to fit the needs of any service area.[3]

Key Issues and Challenges in Competence Assessment

Because the Joint Commission standards for competence assessment were only introduced to the home care field in 1995, there is still some confusion about how to comply with certain requirements—especially those that differ from the requirements in other settings such as hospitals. This section presents the most frequently asked questions about compliance with the competency standards for home care and hospice organizations.

Who needs to be assessed?

The competency standards for home care apply only to direct care staff (such as nurses, home health aides, physical therapists, drivers responsible for equipment delivery and set-up) or staff members whose work directly affects patient care (for example, pharmacists, warehouse staff who clean and sort equipment). Such staff members include all full-time employees, those under contract, and volunteers who are involved in patient care or service, as well as staff who work only weekends or evenings. Some organizations have customer service staff who have telephone contact with patients for purposes of support or education; these people qualify as direct care staff.

This differs from the hospital requirements (*Comprehensive Accreditation Manual for Hospitals*), which state that all employees must be assessed for competencies.

What competencies should be evaluated for supervisors and ancillary staff such as staff development coordinators, team leaders/supervisors, and administrators?

Each organization defines the competencies for all care and service staff members. Competencies for managerial and ancillary staff should be evaluated according to any care/service these staff members may deliver. For example, team leaders or supervisors might be responsible for starting IVs, obtaining lab work via venipunctures, and inserting foley catheters; thus, they would be assessed for competence in these areas. An administrator who has no patient contact and is not responsible for assessing the skills of staff who provide care would not be assessed for any clinical competencies.

How should contract staff be assessed? What is required for on-site personnel records for contract staff?

Contract staff who provide care to patients need to be assessed just as other patient care employees of the organization do. Assessments may be done by the contracted organization (based on the competencies defined by the contracting organization) and then reviewed by the home care organization to ensure that its competency criteria are met, or the home care organization may have contracted staff go through its own competence assessment program. For example, a hospital's competence assessment for a respiratory therapist who works at the hospital two days a week may be accepted by a home care organization if both organizations define the competencies in the same way and *use the same methodology to assess them*.

Organizations are not required to maintain on-site personnel records for contract staff, but at the time of survey, the Joint Commission will request that the organization provide evidence of competence assessment requirements for contract staff (evidence of licensure, orientation, initial and ongoing competence assessments, in-services, health requirements). Organizations should work with their surveyors to determine the most efficient way to review such information.

Are age-specific competencies required?

Home care does not use the term *age-specific*. However, competencies are required as they apply to the individual employee's job and the organization's case mix. For example, an organization that provides home neonatal and pediatric services would be expected to define and assess relevant competencies for staff providing care to these patients. The competencies do not have to be broken down by age group unless the organization chooses to do so.

Do all staff need to be evaluated through observation, or can competence be assessed through other methods such as a written exam or a self-assessment?

Self-assessment alone cannot be used as a validation of competence, but written examination may be an effective way to validate some competencies. For example, confirming that a nurse understands signs and symptoms of hypoglycemia could be accomplished through a written test. However, some processes, such as venipuncture for registered nurses and bathing technique for home health aides, compounding procedures for pharmacists, and correct cleaning of medical equipment by HME staff, require direct observation of skills for proper assessment.

What needs to be assessed through observation?

Not every competency for every position needs to be observed: the organization must determine those that cannot be evaluated properly except by observation, as well as how that observation will take place. This may not have to be done through home visits; some competencies could be observed in the office setting.

Who can assess competence? What if there is no one else on staff who is qualified to assess a specific individual? For example, can a registered nurse evaluate a therapist in a small agency?

The organization should first define the competencies to be evaluated for the staff member. A supervisor or member of another department might be qualified to assess general competencies: the registered nurse may be able to evaluate the therapist's competence in infection control procedures, care coordination, or patient education. For specific clinical or treatment competencies, the organization may have to make arrangements with the nearest hospital, professional organization, home care or hospice organization, or medical university with corresponding programs to arrange for ways to assess competence (a registered nurse would generally not be qualified to assess the skills specific to a therapist's unique scope of practice). This may include developing assessment tools that can be used at the facility, coordinating home visits with a staff member, or reviewing documentation (when appropriate).

How often is assessment required? Is competence testing for all skills required annually?

The frequency of assessment is left up to the individual organization, within the limitations of applicable law and regulation. To determine how frequently staff members need to be evaluated, leaders may ask whether their staff are delivering care to high-risk or problem-prone patients or whether they are working with high-tech equipment that may change and require new training periodically. Also, whenever new services are added to an organization's scope of services, new competencies must be determined as well. Assessments of some (but not necessarily all) competencies must be performed at least once every three years.

Can staff perform tasks in which they have not been deemed "competent"?

Staff members should be deemed competent to perform all skills that may be required according to their job description, education, training, and experience, as well as the organization's scope of services. Competence does not need to be validated before hiring, but it must be validated before the staff member provides care or services.

If confirmation of an employee's competence has been accepted from a previous employer, how can his or her qualifications be verified by the hiring organization?

Organizations need to define the competencies they require for all patient care staff and which of these competencies must be observed. If an individual's competence was assessed by another organization whose requirements correspond (in both definition and methodology) and are acceptable to the hiring organization, the previous competencies may be accepted. To verify competence, the hiring organization may conduct and document a telephone interview with the previous employer or request written verification detailing that employer's assessment.

Can competencies such as peripheral IV insertion, foley catheter insertion, and tracheostomy changes be demonstrated in a lab setting?

The standards permit competencies to be assessed in a lab setting (defined as a "non-patient care setting") if the setting is appropriate to evaluate the defined skill and the organization has defined how the competencies are to be evaluated in such a setting (for example, whether a mannequin or an individual other than a patient may be used). Lab settings may not be appropriate or adequate for evaluating certain skills, such as IV insertion, tracheostomy changes, and foley catheter insertion, which cannot be demonstrated on nonpatients.

How does an organization demonstrate compliance with the competency standards? Is documentation needed?

During the surveys, the surveyor reviews personnel files for evidence of licensure and certification, references, documented experience, and completed competence review forms. The surveyor also observes home visits and interviews the patient/family and the staff member. The important thing is that evidence of qualifications, continued education, and demonstrated competence commensurate with the organization's requirements is present, either in educational records or in personnel records. Organizations should be able to track for individual employees the education and competence assessments required by the organization. (Group attendance records make it difficult to see that an employee has received education and demonstrated competence in specific areas.)

Evidence of the competence assessment program needs to be documented, although the Joint Commission standards do not specify a format that must be used. Surveyors evaluate the program by looking at the written plan leaders formulated originally and by talking with leaders to determine how the plan was developed (how they chose competencies, the ways and times they would be assessed, and the evidence that would be used). Competencies may change over time.

Is it adequate to verify the competence of PICU/NICU nurses based on full-time employment at the home care agency and moonlighting status in high-tech pediatric care? Does the home care organization need to assess competence separately?

Standards require that organizations define the competencies required for staff during the orientation process and on an ongoing basis. During the initial and ongoing assessment process, an organization might define and accept the work experience of PICU/NICU nurses. However, requiring two years experience in a PICU is a qualification, not a competency requirement. The organization would need to determine what competencies the nurses have obtained from their PICU experience and take them into consideration when defining the competencies to be observed during orientation and ongoing assessment. If the final list of competencies includes areas assessed by observation rather than experience, the home care organization would need to observe those skills.

How do the performance improvement requirements fit in?

The performance improvement standards require that organizations collect, analyze, and trend data; the management of human resources standards require that this be done for staff competence. This information is used as the basis for determining staff's learning needs and for developing and improving an effective competence assessment program for the organization.

Summary

An effective competence assessment program must include three basic elements: planning, assessment, and staff development. It is important to note that these steps are not discrete or finite; they are interconnected. Planning lays the groundwork for the assessment process. Assessment is ongoing and shows what training and skills development employees require. Educational programs based on assessment help staff members to improve and may indicate additional areas that need to be addressed in revised planning. The interrelatedness of competence assessment and continuous improvement efforts are discussed further in Chapter 2.

References

1. Benefield LE: Productivity in home health care: Assessing nurse effectiveness and efficiency. Part One. *Home Healthc Nurse* 14(9): 700–702, 1996.

2. Robinson SA and Barberis-Ryan C: Competence assessment: A systematic approach. *Nurs Manage* 26:40, Feb 1995.

3. Byrum CD, Rudisill PT, Singletary MB: The Traveling Salvation Show: A performance-centered skill fair. *J Nurs Staff Dev* 12:198–203, 1996.

CHAPTER 2

For readers whose organizations have not been surveyed in several years, the current survey process may seem a bit different from past surveys. The new survey process has been designed to support patient-centered, performance-focused, functional orientation of the standards in the *Comprehensive Accreditation Manual for Home Care (CAMHC)*. Instead of evaluating specific departments and services, the survey process now concentrates on how various disciplines and staff work together to perform functions that are important to the patient. As a result, surveyors tend to spend less time reviewing paperwork and more time talking with leaders and staff, making home visits, and generally encouraging participation by all health care professionals and patients/families in the process.

Integrating Competence Assessment and Performance Improvement

Obviously, the best way for an organization to implement an effective competence assessment program, maintain accreditation, and prepare for upcoming surveys is to incorporate the standards requirements into its daily operations. As stated in Chapter 1, the standards provide a framework on which to build a competence assessment program. This program is important, not simply because it is required for accreditation, but because it helps organizations ensure that they have competent staff who provide high-quality care.

The cycle for improving performance developed by the Joint Commission integrates a number of different approaches to performance improvement and presents the basic stages in a flexible format that is easy to incorporate into day-to-day operations (See Figure 2-1 page 21). Designed as a continuous and systematic process, it involves four key activities:

1. Design a process;

2. Measure its effectiveness by gathering data for assessment;

3. Assess the data to determine quality of performance; and

4. Improve the process as necessary.

This cycle is echoed in the requirements for the overall competence assessment program:

1. The program is developed initially based on the organization's mission, leaders' and supervisors' expertise, research and benchmarking data, and so on. Competencies are identified for each patient care staff member.

2. Data are gathered through competence assessment, self-assessment, and other tools. They are then aggregated for all employees within a specific category.

3. The aggregated data are analyzed and trended (recorded over time to show trends) to identify staff learning needs and indicate where resources are needed to improve programs such as orientation.

4. Leaders use this information to improve the competence assessment program and corresponding staff development programs. For example, by identifying areas in which staff competence is lower than expected or required, leaders can plan appropriate in-services and prioritize resource use to implement these plans as part of organizationwide planning and performance improvement activities.

Using this model and integrating assessment activities with those for organizationwide performance improvement can be an excellent way to build an effective competence assessment program that

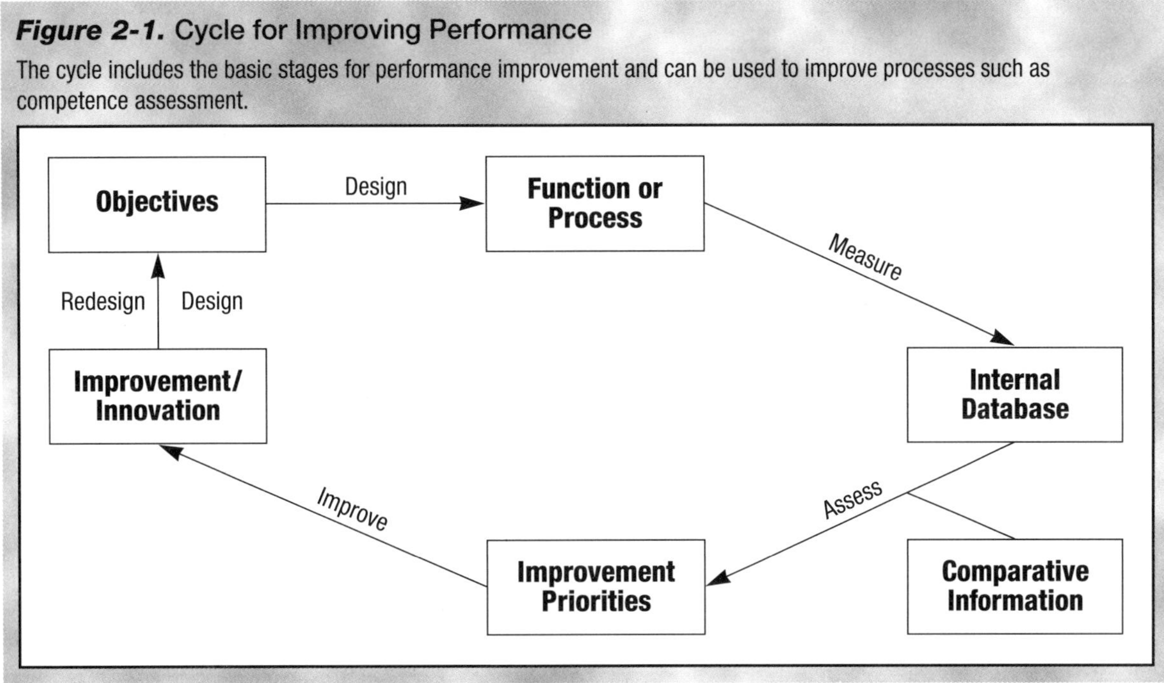

Figure 2-1. Cycle for Improving Performance

The cycle includes the basic stages for performance improvement and can be used to improve processes such as competence assessment.

also meets accreditation requirements. However, it is important to remember that, although an ongoing competence assessment program is necessary for meeting Joint Commission standards, its ultimate advantage (similar to that of the overall performance improvement program) is the resulting increase in staff skills and satisfaction leading to better quality care and service for the patients served.

The Home Care Survey Process

In general terms, surveys consist of preliminary activities, on-site assessment, document and record review, off-site assessment, and other survey activities. The preliminary activities include the presurvey telephone call and the opening conference. On-site assessment consists of a tour of the facility; an evaluation of the organization's performance improvement program; leadership, clinical supervisor, and patient care staff interviews; and telephone calls to patients, staff, and contracted organizations, when appropriate. During document and record review, the surveyor looks at policies and procedures, home care records, personnel records, and other documents, including the organization's education and competence assessment program. Off-site assessment activities comprise home visits, site review of contracted services (if applicable), surveys of branch or warehouse locations (if applicable), staff interviews, and a test of the on-call system. Finally, other survey activities include daily briefings, public information interviews, an education conference, and a leadership exit conference with the organization's leaders to discuss the survey and preliminary findings.

The survey is conducted by one or more surveyors with home care experience appropriate to the organization's services (for example, a pharmacist would survey a home care pharmacy, a registered nurse would survey a home health or hospice organization).

Competence assessment is evaluated in the following survey activities as part of the management of human resources function:

- Leadership interviews;

- Clinical supervisor interviews;

- Patient care staff interviews;

- Document review;

- Personnel record review;

- Test of the on-call system;

- Home visits;

- Survey of branch locations (if applicable); and

- Review of contracted services (if applicable).

The following sections briefly describe these activities and how competence assessment is surveyed.

Leadership Interviews

The surveyor meets with at least one member of the governing body as well as one of the organization's senior leaders during these interviews. Their purpose is to evaluate compliance with standards for improving organization performance and leadership functions and to assess leaders' participation in organizational processes, such as strategic planning, budgeting, prioritization, and resource allocation. The surveyor will ask about how the organization plans for adequate numbers of competent staff. Leaders should be able to show how the competence assessment program was integrated with the organizationwide strategic plan, how time and resources have been budgeted for assessment and staff development, and how the program fits into the organization's priorities.

Some questions the surveyor may ask, based on the standards, include the following:

- Describe your role in recruiting and hiring qualified staff. How does your organization recognize staff achievements? What steps do you take to retain staff and encourage their self-development?

- What kinds of aggregate or trend reports do you receive regarding staff competence? How often are they provided? How are they used?

Clinical Supervisor Interviews

The surveyor meets with supervisory staff to evaluate their roles in planning and directing patient care, including such functions as patient rights; patient care, treatment, and service; education; continuum of care and services; information management; management of human resources; and improving organization performance. The discussion will address the supervisors' role in developing a competence assessment program; identifying competencies for assessment; and hiring, training, and assessing patient care staff.

Some questions the surveyor may ask, based on the standards, include the following:

- How do you train staff who perform waived laboratory testing? How do they demonstrate competence?

- Describe your organization's competence assessment process for various categories of patient care staff (staff nurse, staff pharmacist, HME delivery personnel, hospice bereavement counselor, occupational therapist, home health aide)? What skills do you assess? How often? What happens if someone is deemed incompetent in performing a particular skill?

- Describe your process for ongoing staff development and education. How does the work environment support staff development?

- Describe the orientation process for all staff for whom you are responsible.

- Describe the in-service education process for all staff. Who developed the programs and materials? How were the topics chosen? How do these topics relate to staff competence assessment?

Patient Care Staff Interviews

Patient care staff are interviewed throughout the survey to assess communication between staff, leaders, other health care providers, and patients/families and to evaluate how patient care functions are implemented. The main objectives for competence assessment are verification that assessment takes place, identification of who performs assessments, and initial and ongoing education and training that are made available to staff.

Some questions the surveyor may ask, based on the standards, include the following:

- What are your background, education, and experience relative to your job responsibilities in home care or hospice?

- Describe the orientation you received when you joined this organization.

- How were you evaluated at the end of orientation?

- Are you competent to perform all your duties? How do you know? Has anyone ever evaluated this?

- Give some examples of the education and training you have received since orientation. How often does this generally occur?

- How often are you observed providing care or services connected to care? Who observes you?

- Describe how your organization has assessed your competency.

Document Review

In addition to the review of written policies and procedures, home care records, and personnel records, the document review session allows the surveyor to examine other documentation relating to career services being provided. Competence-related documents in this category would include the following:

- Defined qualifications, competencies, and health status for all levels of staff and volunteers— information that might be found in job descriptions;

- Appropriate documentation for each staff member and supervisor (as required by law and regulation), including current licensure, certification, or registration; education and training; compliance with current health requirements; and knowledge and experience appropriate for assigned responsibilities;

- Documentation of staff attendance at orientation, ongoing education, training, and in-service programs;

- Education plans (if applicable);

- Documentation of competence assessments for each staff member; and

- Staff competence data that have been aggregated and analyzed to assess competence and identify training needs.

Personnel Record Review

The surveyor reviews a sample of personnel files, including full-time and part-time employees and volunteers. The purpose of this activity is to assess the organization's processes for orienting new employees and providing continuing education to staff; defining staff qualifications; selecting, hiring, and training new employees; and assessing and maintaining employee competence.

Some issues the surveyor may address, based on the standards, include the following:

- Is there evidence that the organization has verified each employee's education, training, and (when applicable) current licensure/certification/registration? Is this information up to date?

- Has each employee gone through a staff-orientation process that provides initial job training and information, including an initial assessment of his or her ability to perform specific job responsibilities? Is this documented?

- How was each employee's competence tested (for example, precepted observations, skills lab) before providing patient care and on an ongoing basis as appropriate?

- Is there a process to ensure that each staff member participates in ongoing in-service education sessions and other related training to increase his or her knowledge? Where is this documented?

Test of On-Call System

The purpose of this activity is to determine the accessibility and responsiveness of the organization's after-hours on-call system and to evaluate how patients may obtain medical advice or treatment, equipment support, pharmaceuticals, and so forth in an emergency situation. The test may take place at any time after hours during the course of the survey, and the surveyor uses whatever process the organization has defined for its patients to contact the staff member on call.

Questions asked during this activity relating to competence assessment may include those listed for patient care staff interviews as well as the following:

- What are your responsibilities related to patient care or service?

- What orientation did you receive regarding the on-call system and how to respond to patients' calls? Has someone from the organization tested the system while you were on call?

Home Visits

The surveyor accompanies staff from various disciplines or services on visits to patients' homes (private, residential dwellings or, in the case of hospice patients, a nursing home where the patient lives). The purpose of home visits is to assess the organization's processes related to all patient care functions and to verify staff competence and level of knowledge.

In addition to observing staff members delivering actual care or services, the surveyor will interview patients and their families. These interviews help to verify competency in areas like patient education. For example, the surveyor may ask:

- What have you been taught about the side effects of the medications you're taking? Do you know why you are taking this medication?

- What did the organization's staff teach you about using your equipment (for example, oxygen, Hoyer lift, infusion device) safely and correctly?

- What has the occupational therapist taught you about using adaptive equipment in preparing your meals?

- Has anyone ever accompanied [staff member's name] on a visit?

Survey of Branch Locations

The scope of the survey includes all eligible branch locations or sites of care, including those the surveyor does not visit on site. Branches to be visited are determined before the survey, and on-site visits typically consist of a tour of the facilities, supervisory and staff interviews, at least one home visit for each branch, and home care record review. When the surveyor does not physically visit a branch or care site, it may be included in the survey in several ways, including

- a home visit to or telephone interview with a patient receiving care or service from that location;

- review of a sample of clinical records and personnel files from each location; and

- clinical supervisor and patient care staff interviews at the main office or by telephone.

The surveyor addresses the same topics of staff competence (described previously under specific survey activities) for all branches and care sites.

Review of Contracted Services

Contracted staff are included in the survey of competence assessment just as regular organization staff are. The survey activities involving contract staff include clinical supervisor interviews, patient care staff interviews, personnel record review, document review, and home visits.

In performing these activities, the surveyor concentrates on how and for what competencies contracted staff are assessed. If competence for contracted staff members is assessed by the organization being surveyed, the surveyor checks that they have been evaluated for the same competencies using the same methodology applied to organization staff who provide comparable care or services. If the organization has accepted evaluations of competence from another facility, the surveyor compares the defined competencies and assessment methodologies of the two organizations to be sure the evaluations address (at least) what the surveyed organization addresses for its own staff.

After the Survey

The survey findings are aggregated and reviewed at the Joint Commission headquarters, the decision rules are applied, and the accreditation decision itself is then made. If the decision falls within established parameters, the Joint Commission notifies the organization directly with the decision. Occasionally, accreditation findings that raise special issues are reviewed by the Joint Commission's Accreditation Committee, which then reaches a final decision.

Home care professionals should find that the revised survey process has a number of benefits, including more interaction between surveyors and providers, improved coordination between the organization and the Joint Commission, enhanced education about performance and standards, and a more realistic view of the entire integrated organization. Although the survey still includes review of relevant documents, it emphasizes ongoing discussion between providers and surveyors that shows effective interdisciplinary performance of patient-focused and organization functions.

CHAPTER 3

This chapter presents examples of how home care and hospice organizations can demonstrate compliance with the various standards pertaining to competence assessment. The chapter is not meant to be an exhaustive catalogue of assessment techniques or of methods to comply with the standards. Rather, these examples are intended to generate ideas about how to better plan, implement, and document a competence assessment program and to show how to make these activities known to surveyors.

It is important to remember that documentation is a way to plan, record, and trend results from competence activities, but it is *not* the competence assessment itself, which involves the interplay between the staff member and the individual making the assessment, as well as the patient when direct patient care is assessed. Such interaction is greatly assisted by written instructions and plans. Readers should also note that documentation is only one facet of demonstrating compliance. As discussed in Chapter 2, interviews and discussions are also important parts of Joint Commission surveys.

These examples are not required or endorsed by the Joint Commission for all organizations. They were chosen to illustrate the efforts of a wide variety of home care and hospice organizations. As such, some may not be appropriate for or applicable to all organizations. The examples have been reviewed by Joint Commission staff, surveyors, and customers. The examples themselves have *not* been revised—with the exception of minor editorial corrections or changes—by the Joint Commission.

The examples have been divided into the following sections:

- **Planning for competent staff.** These examples include organizations' development plans, inventories of competencies, and other tools and procedures used to establish a competence assessment program.

- **Assessing individual competence.** This section presents examples of assessment tools from a wide variety of organizations, covering many different types of positions.

- **Maintaining and improving staff competence.** This section includes tools for gathering data related to staff competence, staff education materials, and policies and procedures for ongoing evaluation of proficiency.

Please keep in mind that these examples are, by necessity, excerpts. Each example represents only a part of an organization's efforts; in some cases, only a small portion of a process or tool is presented. Each example illustrates a particular facet of competence assessment. On the whole, however, the examples highlight a broad range of methods for meeting Joint Commission competency standards.

List of Examples

Section 1: Planning for Competent Staff

The examples in this section address matters such as development of assessment programs, definition of competencies and qualifications for various types of patient care staff, and identification of acceptable levels of competence.

Example 1-1. Development Materials for a Competence Assessment Program for Cardiac Home Health Nurses

The position description for Saint Luke's Health System includes the organization's mission, case mix, and core values. Each of these elements was taken into account in the development of the cardiac competency program for Home Health Saint Luke's cardiac home health nurses.

Home Health of Saint Luke's Hospital
Cardiac Competency Program

Developed February 1997

Saint Luke's Health System

Position Description

Mission Statement

The mission of Saint Luke's Health System is to ensure the highest levels of excellence in providing health care services to all patients in a caring environment.

Position Title: Registered Nurse Case Manager   ☐ Saint Luke's Hospital

Job Code: ☐ Crittenton

Department/Cost Center: Home Health   ☐ Saint Luke's Northland

Cost Center Number: 56121   ☐ Ambulatory Care

☒ Home Health

Completed by:

☐ New Position

☒ Revisions to Existing Description   Status: ☒ Exempt   ☐ Nonexempt

(Assigned by Human Resources)

Position Summary

Primary Purpose

This section provides a brief description of the position.

> To prescribe, delegate and coordinate the nursing care provided to assigned patients, pursuant with the goals, objectives, policies and procedures of HHSLH.

(continued on next page)

Example 1-1 (continued). Development Materials for a Competence Assessment
Program for Cardiac Home Health Nurses

Saint Luke's Health System

Position Description

Ages of Patients Served

Please check the appropriate box(es) below to identify the age group(s) of patients served, the nature of services provided and the skills necessary to provide the care appropriate for the ages of the patients served by this position
based upon the position's scope of practice.

Ages of Patients Served	Assessment Diagnostic Testing	Care/Treatment
Neonate	☒	☒
Pediatric	☒	☒
Adolescent	☒	☒
Adult	☒	☒
Geriatric	☒	☒

☐ Does not have clinical responsibilities.

Organizational Relationships

Complete the organizational chart shown below for this position.

Show in detail the organizational structure above and below this position. Identify each position or group of positions
by job title and number of incumbents.

3rd Reporting Level

President/CEO Home Health Services

2nd Reporting Level

Director Home Health Services

1st Reporting Level

Nurse Manager

Other positions reporting to the 1st reporting level

		Registered Nurse Case Manager		

Positions and number of incumbents reporting to this position

(continued on next page)

Example 1-1 (continued). Development Materials for a Competence Assessment Program for Cardiac Home Health Nurses

Saint Luke's Health System

Position Description

Primary Contacts

Identify the **primary** *internal* and *external* contacts and the nature/degree of contacts. The nature of internal contacts is **sharing** information regarding activities or decisions, **influencing** others to act in a manner consistent with the health system objectives, or **directing** and/or integrating the plans, activities or decisions of others. The nature of external contacts is **providing information** or promoting the health system or its products/services or **negotiating** contracts, settlements, etc.

Contacts	Nature/Degree of Contacts
Patients/Families	Direct Care, education
Physicians	Obtain orders and communicate plan of care
Health Team Members	Communicates patient care with PT, ST, OT, MSW and HCA
Community Agencies/Resources	Give referrals, obtain information

Core Value: *Quality/Excellence*

Shared Expectations:

- Strives to be the best; stretches own capabilities to continuously improve. Sets a positive example for others.

- Demonstrates professionalism and accountability.

- Takes initiative to identify and analyze problems; generates alternative solutions. Takes appropriate risks that lead to improved work practices.

- Demonstrates and promotes high standards for quality and productivity; focuses on results.

Position-Specific Accountabilities:

1. Participates in office activities as needed to improve organization flow and effect positive outcomes on patient care.

2. Assists in development of new forms and policies/procedures related to patient care and serves on committees as needed.

3. Promotes the HHA's standard of excellence with physicians and other community organizations.

4. Participates in skills competency testing and keeps current with CEU and CPR certification.

Competencies (the necessary knowledge, skills, behaviors, judgment and personal characteristics required of the position):

1. Demonstrates knowledge of safety requirements, OSHA guidelines and bag technique.

2. Demonstrates knowledge of patient assessment skills.

3. Exhibits knowledge of current nursing standards of practice.

4. Demonstrates ability to plan realistic and individualized patient care.

5. Documents patient care management in accordance with accepted guidelines.

(continued on next page)

Example 1-1 (continued). Development Materials for a Competence Assessment Program for Cardiac Home Health Nurses

---

Saint Luke's Health System

Position Description

Core Value: *Resource Management*

Shared Expectations:

- Examines existing processes and problems and continuously looks for ways to do things better.

- Uses resources (people, supplies, environmental, time) in a responsible cost-effective manner.

- Is fiscally responsible and suggests cost-saving measures.

Position-Specific Accountabilities:

1. Actively participates in cost containment efforts.

2. Demonstrates proper use and maintenance of equipment and supplies.

3. Makes referrals to other services as needs are identified.

Competencies (the necessary knowledge, skills, behaviors, judgment and personal characteristics required of the position):

1. Demonstrates knowledge of correct patient billing for medical supplies.

2. Demonstrates good time management skills.

3. Plans daily route in care delivery to minimize mileage costs.

Core Value: *Customer Focus*

Shared Expectations:

- Treats others with courtesy and respect.

- In partnership with our internal/external customer, identifies expectations and work to meet and exceed them.

- Puts customers first and is responsive to customer requests.

- Maintains a high degree of ethics, integrity, confidentiality.

Position-Specific Accountabilities:

1. Demonstrates knowledge of patients' rights, confidentiality, and privacy.

2. Demonstrates professional attitude and appearance in interactions with patients and other members of the health care team.

3. Responds promptly to patient and family requests.

Competencies (the necessary knowledge, skills, behaviors, judgment and personal characteristics required of the position):

1. Maintains good professional working relationship with physicians and other health care workers.

2. Provides patients with correct information regarding right to privacy and proper grievance procedures.

(continued on next page)

Example 1-1 (continued). Development Materials for a Competence Assessment Program for Cardiac Home Health Nurses

Saint Luke's Health System

Position Description

Core Value: *Teamwork*

Shared Expectations:

- Adjusts and is flexible to meet changing work needs and demands.

- Works cooperatively with own and other teams to achieve common goals.

- Communicates effectively and shares information and resources appropriately.

- Participates in and supports team activities.

- Recognizes others' accomplishments, provides feedback, and mentors others.

Position-Specific Accountabilities:

1. Recognizes each discipline's valuable contribution by promoting interdisciplinary communication and problem solving.

2. Participates in ongoing teaching and training of HHA personnel.

3. Assumes responsibility for appropriate share of the work; modifies own goals to achieve group goals.

4. Serves as a resource or preceptor to other agency employees as requested.

Competencies (the necessary knowledge, skills, behaviors, judgment and personal characteristics required of the position):

1. Collaborates on patient care with other disciplines through case conference, telephone or by written memo.

2. Mentors new employees and students as requested.

3. Participates in team meetings, individual conferences and on planning committees.

Knowledge and Skill

EDUCATION

This section identifies both the **required** and **preferred** level of education for the position.

> **Required**—The level required to meet the minimum qualifications of the position.
> **Preferred**—The ideal level one would seek in recruiting candidates for this position.

Education	Required	Preferred
High school diploma or equivalent	☒	☐
Junior college/Technical school	☒	☐
Bachelor's degree	☐	☒
Master's degree	☐	☐
Ph.D.	☐	☐
M.D.	☐	☐

(continued on next page)

Example 1-1 (continued). Development Materials for a Competence Assessment Program for Cardiac Home Health Nurses

Saint Luke's Health System

Position Description

Knowledge and Skill (continued)

CERTIFICATION/REGISTRATION

This section identifies both the **required** and **preferred** specialized type of licensure, registration, or certification for the position.

> **Required**—The level legally required by the applicable state law to meet the minimum qualifications of the position.
> **Preferred**—The ideal level one would seek in recruiting candidates for this position.

Certification/Registration	Required	Preferred
Kansas state nursing license	☒	☐
Missouri state nursing license	☒	☐
CPR certification	☒	☐
Current driver's license	☒	☐
Automobile collision and liability insurance	☒	☐

EXPERIENCE

This section specifies both the **minimum** and **preferred** level of previous position-related experience to perform the duties. This includes both experience acquired at Saint Luke's and elsewhere.

Experience	Minimum	Preferred
No Previous Experience is Required	☐	☐
Up to 1 Year Experience is Required	☒	☐
1 to 2 Years of Position-Related Experience	☐	☒
2 to 5 Years of Position-Related Experience	☐	☐
5+ Years of Position-Related Experience	☐	☐

The kind of position-related experience includes: Nursing background in med/surg or acute care required, previous experience in home care preferred.

Approvals

Department Head	Date
Administrator	Date
Human Resources	Date

This position description indicates the general nature and level of work experience expected of the position holder. It is not designed to cover or contain a comprehensive listing of activities, duties or responsibilities required of the incumbent.

(continued on next page)

Example 1-1 (continued). Development Materials for a Competence Assessment Program for Cardiac Home Health Nurses

Home Health of Saint Luke's

Cardiac Competency Program

Standard	Teaching/Assessment Method	Reference
The cardiac home health nurse will be able to:		
1. Perform a complete physical assessment, including thorough cardiovascular assessment.	1. AJN Cardiovascular assessment video/Test	1. Appendix 1
2. Demonstrate effective problem solving skills utilizing critical thinking skills for common cardiac problems encountered in the home.	2. Vignettes/Case scenario	2. Appendix 2
3. Describe the Medicare/Medicaid coverage of service guidelines for nursing, therapy, social services, aides and equipment as it pertains to cardiac home care.	3. Self study/Test	3. Appendix 3
4. Describe three indicators for referral of the cardiac patient to other home health services including therapy, home health aide, and hospice.	4. Preceptor interview	4. Appendix 4
5. Deliver care to the general home health cardiac patient, including the CHF, MI, ICD, and post cardiothoracic surgery patient according to professional nursing standards and Agency policy.	5. Video/Test vignettes	5. Appendix 5
6. Complete the outcomes monitoring database correctly and describe objectives and time frames for data collection.	6. Perform with preceptor-record review	6. Appendix 6
7. Describe the components of the Patient Cardiac Home Care Notebook and instruct the patient regarding this resource and utilization.	7. Preceptor observation	7. Appendix 7
8. Describe patient education resources which are available for the cardiac patient.	8. Preceptor interview	8. Appendix 8
9. Verbalize and demonstrate appropriate referral process to outpatient cardiac rehab.	9. Preceptor interview and observation	9. Appendix 9
10. Demonstrate correct use of the CADD pump including operating and evaluating problems.	10. Video demonstration	10. Appendix 10
11. Demonstrate correct administration of intravenous diuretic.	11. Preceptor interview and observation	11. Appendix 11
12. Demonstrate correct technique for central line dressing change.	12. Demonstration	12. Appendix 12

(continued on next page)

Example 1-1 (continued). Development Materials for a Competence Assessment Program for Cardiac Home Health Nurses

Home Health of Saint Luke's

Cardiac Competency Program

Standard	Teaching/Assessment Method	Reference
13. Verbalize care and education given to patients with central line.	13. Preceptor interview	13. Appendix 13
14. Verbalize and demonstrate care of the patient receiving intravenous inotropes.	14. Vignettes/Preceptor observation	14. Appendix 14
15. Demonstrate use of the Propac monitor.	15. Demonstration	15. Appendix 15
16. Accurately identify basic heart rhythms.	16. ECG interpretation and recognition of dysrhythmias test	16. Appendix 16
17. Verbalize appropriate use of ace inhibitors, antiarrythmics, beta blockers, calcium channel blockers, diuretics, vasodilators, inotropes and discuss side effects, contraindications, dosing, schedule, and laboratory recommendations of each.	17. Self study/Test and preceptor interview	17. Appendix 17
18. Describe the management principles of anti-coagulation therapy in the home.	18. Self study/Test	18. Appendix 18
19. Verbalize cardiac on-call procedure.	19. Preceptor/Nurse manager interview	19. Appendix 19

Source: Kathy M. Noland, RN, PhD, President, Saint Luke's Shawnee Mission System Home Care Services, Kansas City, MO.

Example 1-2. Job Description and Competencies for Oxygen Technicians

Here, the key duties or responsibilities listed in the job description for oxygen technicians are identified first. Performance standards are then defined for the same categories. Finally, a checklist is used for assessment of identified competencies based on the job description and performance standards.

Job Title: Oxygen Technicians

Department: Home Oxygen/DME

Supervisor: Home Oxygen Director

Job Summary:

Under the supervision of the Hospice/Home Oxygen Director, the Oxygen Technician receives oxygen DME orders, coordinates oxygen set-up, delivery, maintenance, and supplies to patients homes. Maintains all oxygen equipment and supplies. Patient population served is neonate through geriatric.

Key Duties:

Equipment Maintenance:

1. Checks all equipment according to the maintenance schedule as suggested by the manufacturer.

2. Repairs all equipment.

3. Documents all scheduled and nonscheduled equipment maintenance.

4. Checks and records the oxygen contents as defined in the Policy and Procedure Manual.

5. Alerts Plant Services Department of any maintenance required by the delivery vehicles.

6. Checks the fluid levels and electrical lighting of the delivery vehicles.

7. Cleans and maintains patient equipment in an aseptic fashion and follows department policy.

Equipment Delivery:

1. Delivers oxygen, durable medical equipment, and supplies to private and commercial accounts.

2. Practices safety in delivery of equipment.

3. Technicians are subject to unusual working conditions during deliveries.

Clerical:

1. Charts patient data, schedules, and appointments, and photocopies and files medical records.

2. Endorses all pick-up slips, delivery slips, Authorization of Insurance Benefits, Wisconsin Power and Light information, Patient Bill of Rights and safety instructions with general information folders, and all equipment maintenance forms.

3. Charts equipment maintenance.

4. Receives new patient data.

5. Charts daily responsibilities and duties.

Home O_2/DME:

1. Follows infection control guidelines as outlined in the Department Policy and Procedure Manual.

2. Visits all oxygen-using patients on a routine basis.

(continued on next page)

Example 1-2 (continued). Job Description and Competencies for Oxygen Technicians

General:

1. Performs equipment cleaning.

2. Participates in "on call" during all non-working hours.

3. Established Daily Work Assignment, ordering inventory supplies and calibration of equipment for Home O_2/DME to accomplish the goals and objectives of the department.

4. Reports any potentially harmful situation to the Director.

5. Communicates with home patients and families about rental and purchased equipment.

6. Relates any harmful or questionable circumstances to the department director.

7. Referral source for other needed services, i.e., home care, hospice, respiratory therapy.

Unusual Working Conditions:

1. Potential exposure to bacterial and viral diseases.

2. "On call" responsibilities may exceed oxygen equipment malfunction in patients' homes.

3. Travel in unusual weather conditions.

Specifications:

1. Education is generally found in four years of high school, equipment and safety seminars, and oxygen repair school.

2. Able to lift 160 lbs.

3. Commercial Drivers License with only one moving violation in two years.

4. Trained in equipment use, cleaning, and maintenance.

5. Ability to understand the patient/client's overall character.

6. An understanding of the limitations of services rendered.

7. An understanding of appropriate resources.

Physical Demands:

Prolonged, extensive, or considerable standing/walking. Lifts, positions, pushes, and/or transfers patients. Lifts supplies/equipment, considerable reaching, stooping, bending, kneeling, and crouching.

Working Conditions:

Contact with patients under wide variety of circumstances. May be exposed to/occasionally exposed to patient elements. Exposed to unpleasant elements (accidents, injuries, and illness). Subject to varying and unpredictable situations. Handles emergency or crisis situations. May work with communicable diseases.

The above statements are intended to describe the general nature and level of work being performed. They are not intended to be construed as an exhaustive list of all responsibilities, duties, and skills required of personnel so classified.

(continued on next page)

Example 1-2 (continued). Job Description and Competencies for Oxygen Technicians

Performance Standards

Job Title: Oxygen Technicians

Department: Home Oxygen/DME

Supervisor: Home Oxygen Director

Key Job Accountability		Performance Standards
Equipment Maintenance	30%	1. Checks all equipment according to the manufacturer's guidelines. 2. Repairs all equipment on as-needed basis. 3. Documents all scheduled and non-scheduled repair/maintenance. 4. Checks and records the oxygen contents as defined in the Policy and Procedure Manual. 5. Alerts Plant Services Department of any maintenance required by the delivery vehicles. 6. Checks and documents the fluid levels and electrical lighting of delivery vehicle daily. 7. Cleans and maintains patient equipment in an aseptic manner and follows department policy. 8. Follows infection control guidelines as outlined in department policy and procedure manual.
Equipment Delivery	30%	1. Creates and updates a delivery listing on a daily basis. Daily updates or initials the priority list for emergency situations. 2. Delivers equipment to clients on a timely basis as scheduled and whenever necessary. 3. Abides by all traffic and governing regulations when driving the delivery vehicles. 4. Practices safety precautions as outlined in the Policy and Procedure Manual. 5. Delivers Home O_2/DME as ordered by a physician and as policy dictates without incident. 6. Visits all oxygen-using patients on routine basis.
Collaboration	20%	1. Charts all appropriate patient data on designated forms, schedules Integration delivery appointments, photocopies and files medical records. 2. Receives new patient data. 3. Endorses and itemizes all pickup and delivery slips. 4. Endorses and files all equipment maintenance forms. 5. POC updated every 30 days. 6. Identifies referrals appropriately. 7. Contacts primary nurse with information obtained through visit.

(continued on next page)

Example 1-2 (continued). Job Description and Competencies for Oxygen Technicians

Performance Standards

Job Title: Oxygen Technicians

Key Job Accountability		Performance Standards
Customer Service	10%	

1. Appearance Standards
   A. Wear appropriate clothing for your department and position.
   B. Wear your name badge at all times.
   C. Be neat and clean.
   D. Avoid excessive makeup, perfume, jewelry.

2. Welcome and Greetings
   A. Speak first with a friendly greeting and a smile.
   B. Use the person's name when possible; don't use first names without permission.
   C. Maintain good eye contact.
   D. Ask open-ended questions.
   E. When talking to or assisting someone, give your full attention to that person; do not interrupt coworkers when they are assisting someone.
   F. When you approach a patient to give care, introduce yourself and tell the person why you are there.

3. Courtesy
   A. Stop personal conversations when a person approaches or state that you will be available to help shortly.
   B. Excuse yourself if you must answer a phone or attend to other business while helping someone.
   C. If you are on the phone when a person approaches, acknowledge his or her presence while completing the call.
   D. When asked a question that you cannot answer, take time to find the answer or direct the person to someone who can help.
   E. Keep visitors or patients informed as to delays.
   F. Make sure the person you are helping has all the necessary information before you send him or her on the way. If the person seems unclear, offer to escort the person or get someone else to do so.
   G. Refrain from criticizing the person who needs your help.
   H. Relay messages to those assuming your responsibilities.

4. Basic Rules
   A. Respect the privacy of others.
   B. Maintain confidentiality at all times.
   C. Never discuss patient cases in public, including hallways, elevators, and cafeteria.
   D. Do not complain or criticize physicians or coworkers.
   E. Do not use profanity, slang, or jargon.

(continued on next page)

Example 1-2 (continued). Job Description and Competencies for Oxygen Technicians

Performance Standards

Job Title: Oxygen Technicians

Key Job Accountability		Performance Standards

Customer Service (continued)	10%	5. Telephone Service
		  A. Telephone calls will be answered within 3 rings.
		  B. When answering internal calls, the employee will identify the Unit or Department and give his or her name.
		  C. Tone of voice will be alert, pleasant, natural and expressive.
		  D. Calls will be screened with the phrase: "May I tell her who is calling?" If the caller asks if the person is in, say "I will check; may I tell him who is calling?"
		  E. The caller's name will be used by the person answering the phone when possible.
		  F. Messages will be taken accurately.
		  G. Telephone message centers will include a list of frequently called numbers, hospital directories for in house, physician's offices, radio pagers, and telephone message pads. Messages should be retrieved and delivered promptly.
		  H. Calls will be terminated courteously.
		  I. Telephone users will not eat or chew gum while using the telephone.
		  J. Telephone users will not carry on other conversations while using the telephone.
		  K. When placing a call, identify yourself when the called department answers.
		  L. Transfer calls promptly.
		  M. If you receive a transferred call by mistake, ask the caller whom he or she is trying to reach and graciously transfer the call to the correct area.
		  N. If you dial a wrong number, don't just hang up.
		  O. Know your department phone numbers and extensions so you can dial direct from the outside.

General	10%	1. Relates any harmful or questionable circumstance to the department supervisor. 2. Attends department meetings 100% of the time unless excused by Director. 3. Knows policies and procedures of the department.

Department Manager: ____   Date: _______________

The above performance standards have been discussed with me.

Employee:____   Date: _______________

(continued on next page)

Example 1-2 (continued). Job Description and Competencies for Oxygen Technicians

Addendum
Home Oxygen Technician (Equipment Handler)

Performance Standards

Key Job Accountability	Does Not Meet Standards	Exceeding Standards
1. Equipment Maintenance	Alerts Plant Services and supervisor of any maintenance required by delivery vehicles 1 day after problem is encountered.	Alerts Plant Services and supervisor on any maintenance required by delivery vehicles immediately when problem is encountered.
	Does not complete concentrator checks every 6 weeks.	Completes concentrator checks no more than or less than monthly.
	Check fluid levels and electrical lighting of delivery vehicle weekly.	Checks fluid levels and electrical lighting of delivery vehicle daily.
	Checks any equipment without review of manufacturer's guidelines.	Checks all equipment with review of manufacturer's guidelines.
	Does not document ALL scheduled and non-scheduled repair/ maintenance.	Documents ALL scheduled and non-scheduled repair/maintenance in detail.
2. Equipment Delivery	Does not communicate patient instructions.	Clearly communicates and observes patient equipment use.
	Delivers equipment and oxygen 1 day after scheduled.	Delivers equipment and oxygen within 10 min. of set time if established.
	Does not communicate with peers regarding schedule.	Does keep in contact 2–3 times per day with peers.
3. Collaboration and Integration	Fills out new data account forms, delivery slips, time sheets and pick-up slips completely only 60% of time.	Fills out new account data forms, delivery slips, pick-up slips, and time sheets completely 95% of time.
	Information not passed to appropriate team members 3 times.	Contacts primary nurse with information obtained through visits and documents such.
		Updates the POC every 30 days.
		Identifies when to refer patients to respiratory therapist or nursing services.
		Contacts Director for clarification.

(continued on next page)

Example 1-2 (continued). Job Description and Competencies for Oxygen Technicians

Oxygen Technician Competency Checklist

Technician name:____

Competency checklist completed by:____

Demonstrates knowledge and competence in: **Date Assessed**

1. Ability to determine the structural requirements for a patient to use oxygen/respiratory equipment (for example, doorway width). _______________

2. Electrical requirements for home oxygen equipment. _______________

3. Environmental requirements (adequate storage space). _______________

4. Arranging home to accommodate equipment's physical, electrical, and other needs. _______________

5. Unpacking, assembling, and performing needed operational checks of equipment. _______________

6. Verifying the appropriate considerations for equipment adaptation. _______________

7. Correctly using, operating, storing, maintaining and cleaning/disinfecting equipment and related supplies in the home, according to manufacturer's guidelines. _______________

8. Checking the safety of all equipment. _______________

9. Having problem identification skills, problem-solving skills and trouble-shooting procedures on all equipment. _______________

10. Having access to appropriate resources (such as supervisory consultation or manufacturer's guidelines) to aid in problem solving and troubleshooting. _______________

11. Using routine response procedures. _______________

12. Using on call or after-hour response procedures. _______________

13. Using emergency response procedures. _______________

14. Making sure that appropriately qualified staff are available to respond to any type of emergency related to the equipment provided. _______________

15. Using appropriate backup systems for patients. _______________

16. Maintaining equipment utilizing appropriate procedures. _______________

17. Current or ongoing education. _______________

Example 1-3. Inventories of Skills and Experience for Nurses in a Private Duty Agency

Based on skill and experience inventories, such as these for registered nurses and licensed practical nurses in a high-tech pediatric private duty agency, leaders can identify which skills require observation and what evidence of competence is acceptable for other skills. In developing tools for inventories, it is important to consider all patient populations served and their specific needs (for example, children's ages and those with special needs such as premature infants).

Pediatric Special Care

RN Skill and Experience Inventory

Name: ____   Date: _______________________

Key: Self Evaluation: (circle one) 1 = experienced, confident 2 = little experience, not confident 3 = not experienced NA = not applicable

1. Knowledge of Nursing Process

a. Health history/Physical exam   1 2 3 NA

b. Developing a problem list   1 2 3 NA

c. Purpose of plan of treatment   1 2 3 NA

d. Assessing patient's response
to treatment   1 2 3 NA

e. Establishing & revising goals   1 2 3 NA

f. Assessing DC planning needs   1 2 3 NA

g. DC instruction   1 2 3 NA

2. Documentation Skills

a. Incident/Variance reporting   1 2 3 NA

b. Narrative clinical notes, flow charts   1 2 3 NA

c. Documenting of verbal orders   1 2 3 NA

3. Plan of Treatment

a. Reviews plan of treatment
prior to care   1 2 3 NA

b. Performs services as ordered   1 2 3 NA

c. Documents according to plan   1 2 3 NA

d. Communicates/Coordinates
if appropriate   1 2 3 NA

4. Effective Case Coordination

a. Reports and documents key
information to or from
parent/caregiver, physician,
clinical nurse manager   1 2 3 NA

b. Reports and documents key
information to or from other team
members (PT, OT, Teacher, DME)   1 2 3 NA

c. Community resources   1 2 3 NA

**5. Medical Equipment Ordering
and Management**   1 2 3 NA

**6. Patient/Client Vulnerability and
Home Safety**   1 2 3 NA

7. Infection Control

a. Handwashing   1 2 3 NA

b. Protective equipment   1 2 3 NA

c. Safe needle technique   1 2 3 NA

d. Exposure plan   1 2 3 NA

e. Equipment care   1 2 3 NA

8. Patient/Client Education

a. Determines learning needs/
Sets objectives   1 2 3 NA

b. Develops/Implements teaching   1 2 3 NA

c. Evaluates effectiveness of
teaching   1 2 3 NA

d. Documents patient/client
response   1 2 3 NA

9. Home Glucose Monitoring

a. Purpose of test   1 2 3 NA

b. Specimen collection   1 2 3 NA

c. Specimen preservation   1 2 3 NA

d. Instrument calibration   1 2 3 NA

e. Quality control mechanism   1 2 3 NA

f. Performance/Interpretation of tests   1 2 3 NA

10. Medications

I. Administration techniques

a. oral   1 2 3 NA

b. rectal   1 2 3 NA

c. IM   1 2 3 NA

d. subcutaneous   1 2 3 NA

e. ear   1 2 3 NA

f. eye   1 2 3 NA

g. intravenous   1 2 3 NA

h. central line (Broviac)   1 2 3 NA

II. Pediatric Safe Dosage Calculations   1 2 3 NA

(continued on next page)

Example 1-3 (continued). Inventories of Skills and Experience for Nurses in a Private Duty Agency

Pediatric Special Care

RN Skill and Experience Inventory

Clinical Skills
1. Principles of aseptic technique   1 2 3 NA
2. Vital Signs/I+0   1 2 3 NA

Respiratory System
1. Respiratory assessment   1 2 3 NA
2. Use and care of oxygen   1 2 3 NA
3. Oral/nasal suctioning   1 2 3 NA
4. Nebulizer mist therapy (NMT)   1 2 3 NA
5. CPT and postural drainage   1 2 3 NA
6. Tracheostomy care   1 2 3 NA
7. Tracheostomy change   1 2 3 NA
8. Tracheostomy suctioning   1 2 3 NA
9. Home ventilator management   1 2 3 NA
    LP6/LP-10   1 2 3 NA
    Bipap to trach   1 2 3 NA
    Bipap to mask   1 2 3 NA
10. Pulse oximetry   1 2 3 NA
11. Apnea monitor   1 2 3 NA
12. Pulmoaide   1 2 3 NA

Cardiovascular
1. Cardiovascular assessment   1 2 3 NA
2. Pulses (apical, radial, femoral, pedial)   1 2 3 NA
3. Edema assessment   1 2 3 NA
4. CPR (infant, child, adult)   1 2 3 NA

Neurologic
1. General exam (pulses, LOC, grasp)   1 2 3 NA
2. Seizure precautions   1 2 3 NA
3. Spinal/head injury care   1 2 3 NA

Gastro-intestinal
1. General exam/auscultation of bowel sounds   1 2 3 NA
2. Abdominal girth   1 2 3 NA
3. Nasogastric tube insertion   1 2 3 NA
4. Gastric tube feedings (G-tube, J-tube)   1 2 3 NA
5. Gastrostomy tube insertion   1 2 3 NA
6. Gastrostomy stoma care   1 2 3 NA
7. Bottle feeding   1 2 3 NA
8. Colostomy stoma care   1 2 3 NA
9. Colostomy irrigation care   1 2 3 NA

Integumentary
1. General exam   1 2 3 NA
2. Sterile dressing change   1 2 3 NA
3. Wet to dry dressing   1 2 3 NA

Genitourinary
1. General exam   1 2 3 NA
2. Urinary catheterization
    female   1 2 3 NA
    male   1 2 3 NA
3. Ileostomy care   1 2 3 NA

Musculoskeletal
1. General exam   1 2 3 NA
2. ROM (active and passive)   1 2 3 NA
3. Cast assessment and care   1 2 3 NA
4. Devices
    Wheelchair   1 2 3 NA
    Hoyer lift   1 2 3 NA

Metabolic
1. Diabetic teaching
    a. Insulin types & administration   1 2 3 NA
    b. Use, care and technique of Glucose Monitoring System   1 2 3 NA
    c. Diet, exercise   1 2 3 NA
    d. S & S of glycemic reactions, skin care   1 2 3 NA

Children's Ages
_____ Neonates/Newborns
_____ Infants
_____ Toddlers
_____ Preschoolers
_____ School age
_____ Adolescent

Special Needs Children
_____ Neurologically impaired
_____ Premature babies
_____ Oxygen dependent
_____ Ventilator dependent
_____ Musculoskeletal degeneration
_____ Seizure disorders
_____ Head/spinal injury

(continued on next page)

Example 1-3 (continued). Inventories of Skills and Experience for Nurses in a Private Duty Agency

Pediatric Special Care

LPN Skill and Experience Inventory

Name: ____ Date: _______________________

Key: Self Evaluation: (circle one) 1 = experienced, confident 2 = little experience, not confident 3 = not experienced NA = not applicable

1. Knowledge of Nursing Process

a. Assisting in the development of a problem list 1 2 3 NA

b. Purpose of plan of treatment 1 2 3 NA

c. Assessing patient's response to treatment 1 2 3 NA

d. Assessing DC planning needs 1 2 3 NA

e. DC instruction 1 2 3 NA

2. Documentation Skills

a. Incident/Variance reporting 1 2 3 NA

b. Narrative clinical notes, flow charts 1 2 3 NA

c. Documenting of verbal orders 1 2 3 NA

3. Plan of Treatment

a. Reviews plan of treatment prior to care 1 2 3 NA

b. Performs services as ordered 1 2 3 NA

c. Documents according to plan 1 2 3 NA

d. Communicates/Coordinates if appropriate 1 2 3 NA

4. Effective Case Coordination

a. Reports and documents key information to or from parent/caregiver, physician, clinical nurse manager 1 2 3 NA

b. Reports and documents key information to or from other team members (PT, OT, Teacher, DME) 1 2 3 NA

c. Community resources 1 2 3 NA

5. Medical Equipment Ordering and Management 1 2 3 NA

6. Patient/Client Vulnerability and Home Safety 1 2 3 NA

7. Infection Control

a. Handwashing 1 2 3 NA

b. Protective equipment 1 2 3 NA

c. Safe needle technique 1 2 3 NA

d. Exposure plan 1 2 3 NA

e. Equipment care 1 2 3 NA

8. Patient/Client Education

a. Determines learning needs/ Sets objectives 1 2 3 NA

b. Develops/Implements teaching 1 2 3 NA

c. Evaluates effectiveness of teaching 1 2 3 NA

d. Documents patient/client response 1 2 3 NA

9. Home Glucose Monitoring

a. Purpose of test 1 2 3 NA

b. Specimen collection 1 2 3 NA

c. Specimen preservation 1 2 3 NA

d. Instrument calibration 1 2 3 NA

e. Quality control mechanism 1 2 3 NA

f. Performance/Interpretation of tests 1 2 3 NA

10. Medications

I. Administration techniques

a. oral 1 2 3 NA

b. rectal 1 2 3 NA

c. IM 1 2 3 NA

d. subcutaneous 1 2 3 NA

e. ear 1 2 3 NA

f. eye 1 2 3 NA

g. intravenous 1 2 3 NA

h. central line (Broviac) 1 2 3 NA

II. Pediatric Safe Dosage Calculations 1 2 3 NA

(continued on next page)

Example 1-3 (continued). Inventories of Skills and Experience for Nurses in a Private Duty Agency

Pediatric Special Care

LPN Skill and Experience Inventory

Clinical Skills

1. Principles of aseptic technique   1 2 3 NA
2. Vital Signs/I+0   1 2 3 NA

Respiratory System

1. Respiratory assessment   1 2 3 NA
2. Use and care of oxygen   1 2 3 NA
3. Oral/nasal suctioning   1 2 3 NA
4. Nebulizer mist therapy (NMT)   1 2 3 NA
5. CPT and postural drainage   1 2 3 NA
6. Tracheostomy care   1 2 3 NA
7. Tracheostomy change   1 2 3 NA
8. Tracheostomy suctioning   1 2 3 NA
9. Home ventilator management   1 2 3 NA
     LP6/LP-10   1 2 3 NA
     Bipap to trach   1 2 3 NA
     Bipap to mask   1 2 3 NA
10. Pulse oximetry   1 2 3 NA
11. Apnea monitor   1 2 3 NA
12. Pulmoaide   1 2 3 NA

Cardiovascular

1. Cardiovascular assessment   1 2 3 NA
2. Pulses (apical, radial, femoral, pedial)   1 2 3 NA
3. Edema assessment   1 2 3 NA
4. CPR (infant, child, adult)   1 2 3 NA

Neurologic

1. General exam (pulses, LOC, grasp)   1 2 3 NA
2. Seizure precautions   1 2 3 NA
3. Spinal/head injury care   1 2 3 NA

Gastro-intestinal

1. General exam/auscultation
     of bowel sounds   1 2 3 NA
2. Abdominal girth   1 2 3 NA
3. Nasogastric tube insertion   1 2 3 NA
4. Gastric tube feedings
     (G-tube, J-tube)   1 2 3 NA
5. Gastrostomy tube insertion   1 2 3 NA
6. Gastrostomy stoma care   1 2 3 NA
7. Bottle feeding   1 2 3 NA
8. Colostomy stoma care   1 2 3 NA
9. Colostomy irrigation care   1 2 3 NA

Integumentary

1. General exam   1 2 3 NA
2. Sterile dressing change   1 2 3 NA
3. Wet to dry dressing   1 2 3 NA

Genitourinary

1. General Exam   1 2 3 NA
2. Urinary catheterization
     female   1 2 3 NA
     male   1 2 3 NA
3. Ileostomy care   1 2 3 NA

Musculoskeletal

1. General exam   1 2 3 NA
2. ROM (active and passive)   1 2 3 NA
3. Cast assessment and care   1 2 3 NA
4. Devices
     Wheelchair   1 2 3 NA
     Hoyer lift   1 2 3 NA

Metabolic

1. Diabetic Teaching
     a. Insulin types & administration   1 2 3 NA
     b. Use, care and technique of
        Glucose Monitoring System   1 2 3 NA
     c. Diet, exercise   1 2 3 NA
     d. S & S of glycemic reactions,
        skin care   1 2 3 NA

Children's Ages

_____ Neonates/Newborns
_____ Infants
_____ Toddlers
_____ Preschoolers
_____ School age
_____ Adolescent

Special Needs Children

_____ Neurologically impaired
_____ Premature babies
_____ Oxygen dependent
_____ Ventilator dependent
_____ Musculoskeletal degeneration
_____ Seizure disorders
_____ Head/spinal injury

Source: Pediatric Special Care, Inc., Troy, MI.

Example 1-4. Competency Inventory for Identifying Staff Needs

This inventory addresses general competencies and can be adapted for any home care professional. It can be used as both an assessment tool and a means of identifying areas in which leaders may wish to institute organizationwide programs for staff development or continuing education.

Yearly Home Services Competency Inventory

Salaried Personnel

Name: _______________

Title: _______________

NA = Not Applicable

R = Routinely Performed
I = Inservice
P = Procedure Reviewed
D = Procedure Demonstrated

Skills	Demo	Return Demo	Competent	Year ___	Year ___	Year ___	Year ___	Year ___	Year ___	Year ___	Year ___
Problem Management											
Conflict Resolution											
Budgeting											
Critical Thinking											
Resource Utilization											
Decision Making											
Team Building											
Risk Management											
Customer Relations											
Performance Evaluation											
Productivity											
Nursing Process											
Communication											
Verbal											
Written											
Time Management											
Delegation											
Managing Priorities											
Managing Change											
Strategic Planning											
Project Management											
Hospitalwide Inservice											
Age-Specific Needs of Population Served											
Received PPD											
OSHA Bloodborne Pathogens											

Source: Reid Hospital and Health Care Services, Home Services Department, Richmond, IN.

Example 1-5. Competence Assessment Program Summary for Staff Providing Care to Ventilator-Dependent Patients

This summary identifies what was taken into consideration during the planning stage for a large home care agency's competence assessment program. It shows the types of knowledge, skills, and abilities that needed to be demonstrated by staff members, as well as what activities and settings would be used for evaluation. Mapping out the program in writing is extremely useful for future reference and review. When and if the organization's mission and/or scope of care and services changes, competencies may change as well.

Competency Program Development
Shands HomeCare, 1994–1996

Premises/Underlying Assumptions/Parameters

1. Program must meet 95 JCAHO HomeCare accreditation standards that mandate competency validation of all direct care staff agencies.

2. Program must also be consistent/congruent with hospital standards of care & practice as well as with competency validation program used by the Department of Nursing & Patient Services. Congruence was required in order to facilitate consistency of care across settings as well as to meet risk management directives and also to give the home care nursing staff credibility in terms of clinical competence and expertise with the hospital's medical and nursing staff.

3. Program must be flexible enough to meet needs of varying business lines (hourly, intermittent, Medicare, "private") while maintaining consistent standards.

4. Program must be designed to permit reasonably rapid hiring/competency validation process to meet needs generated by last minute/unexpected referrals or needs for staff.

5. Cost of program must be managed so that direct & indirect costs of providing services do not increase significantly.

6. Program must address core competencies that cut across all business lines, all agencies regardless of census, types of patients served, or location in the state of Florida (i.e., program must work for all agencies throughout the system).

7. At the same time, program must also allow for differences generated by differences in patient populations and types of care/service provided.

8. Identified competencies must flow from established outcomes. Outcomes may be drawn from home health care licensure & certification regulations as well as from the clinical standards of care and practice related to specialty skills, high tech skills, or management of special patient populations. Outcomes may also be drawn from outcomes identified on specific clinical paths or nursing care plans for groups of patients.

9. Competency is operationally defined as the ability to simultaneously integrate the knowledge, skills, and attitudes required for performance in a designated setting. Involves performance of a task, critical thinking around that task, & interaction with patient during performance of task/care in the actual setting.

10. Since competency is setting dependent, overall competency validation process must include a supervised visit or witnessed ride in which the employee is directly observed when providing care.

Development History

We began our competency development by defining the basic or core competency categories that any RN or LPN practicing in home care needed to meet. The categories included making a home visit, performing basic nursing skills according to agency policy and procedure, following infection control policies and procedures, and completing documentation according to agency standards. The specific competencies and required behaviors were developed by the area executive directors who were in place at the time with input from agency administrators and clinical managers.

(continued on next page)

Example 1-5 (continued). Competence Assessment Program Summary for Staff Providing Care to Ventilator-Dependent Patients

Competency Program Development

Shands HomeCare, 1994–1996

These competencies were defined as the minimum or initial competency requirement that must be met before the new employee could be assigned to see patients independently. It was recommended that the basic competency validation be met PRIOR to employee's participation in specialty orientation programs and specialty competency validations.

The Skilled Nurse Visit (SNV) Form (Attachment A) was developed to document the employee's completion of the competency requirements. To validate these competencies, each new RN/LPN is required to complete a witnessed ride; the new RN/LPN's performance in the home is evaluated against the core competencies by another RN who has already met SNV competency requirements.

In addition to the basic or generic competencies, we developed some specific specialty competency checklists. These checklists are based on our clinical standards, and were developed in collaboration with HomeCare clinical experts from all regions in the state. I've included an excerpt from one clinical standard and the corresponding checklist; please see Attachments B and C. Specialty competency validation must be done before the employee is assigned to provide that specialty care independently in the home setting.

The ongoing competency validation requirement was defined as a minimum of one supervised visit per year using the categories outlined on the Joint Visit Ride Form (See Attachment D). The supervised visit should be done in conjunction with the employee's annual performance appraisal. If the employee is providing specialty services (such as infusion, pediatric, etc.), the supervised visit should be scheduled for a visit that involves performance of that care.

Maintaining the revalidating specialty competencies in agencies where the specialty population is "low volume" have been ongoing challenges. At the time of the performance evaluation, if the nurse cannot be observed providing specialty care due to a lack of appropriate patients, he/she will be directly observed providing that care at the next available opportunity.

The competency categories on Joint Visit Ride Form were drawn from operational policies and clinical standards. These categories reflect core competencies that cut across setting, services, types of patients, and locations.

The supervisor performing the joint visit ride evaluation is expected to evaluate the employee's performance against the relevant established standards. For example, the performance of an RN providing infusion services would be evaluated against the following standards:

- infusion policies and procedures that relate to the specific care he/she is providing at the time of the witnessed ride

- pertinent infection control policies

- clinical standards related to assessment and teaching.

The generic comments section on the form allows the evaluator to comment on the employee's performance specific to specialty standards.

Our goal is to continue to develop clinical standards of practice that can be used to both guide patient care and evaluate staff performance in the care of specific patient populations. We will continue to use the process established by the Department of Nursing and Patient Services and focus heavily on the identification of specific patient outcomes. See Attachment E for an example of a standard including outcomes.

(continued on next page)

Example 1-5 (continued). Competence Assessment Program Summary for Staff Providing Care to Ventilator-Dependent Patients

Competency Program Development

Shands HomeCare, 1994–1996

The steps of our process are as follows:

- First, groups of patients are identified. Patients may be "grouped" on the basis of medical diagnosis, type of therapy, use of a particular kind of equipment, or management of specific common problems (such as neutropenia, etc.).

- Patient outcomes are then identified for a specific group of patients.

- Then, the nursing care or nursing interventions that are indicated to facilitate the patient's achievement of the desired outcomes are identified and outlined.

- Next, the core or key things that the nurse must know and be able to do in order to implement the interventions and facilitate outcome achievement are identified.

- These "key things" form the basis of the required specialty competencies & the requirements for how and when the competencies will be validated.

- Once the required competencies are identified, appropriate educational programming (orientation and inservice) is planned to assist the nurse in meeting and maintaining competencies.

We plan to establish a system to use the data obtained from evaluating the nurse's performance against our established standards to help us meet the JCAHO requirement for aggregate data collection and trending related to competencies.

(continued on next page)

Example 1-5 (continued). Competence Assessment Program Summary for Staff
Providing Care to Ventilator-Dependent Patients

Attachment A

Documentation of Completion of
SNV (Intermittent Visit) Competencies

Name: ____   Date: __________________

Key Behaviors	Date Met/Initials
Competency: Upon completion of orientation, the orientee will complete and document a skilled nurse visit according to agency policy and procedures.	

1. Obtains assignment & report from designated person in office.
   – primary reason for visit
   – overview of patient status
   – reportable signs and symptoms
   – procedures/teaching to be done
   – obtains necessary supplies, chart forms before making visit	

2. Makes skilled nurse visit; complete visit includes
   – collects & documents subjective data from patient and/or caregiver
   – completes and documents assessment; includes
     * vital signs
     * objective data (i.e., physical assessment, observation of performance of skill, etc.)
     * caregiver's limitations & abilities
     * patient's functional limitations
   – implements planned care
   – assesses & documents patient/caregiver's response to care given	

3. Documents visit and patient status on progress note; documentation meets the following criteria:
   – maintains confidentiality
   – avoids value laden phrasing
   – is completed within 24 hours
   – is legible
   – is precise
   – includes signs/symptoms of any changes in patient condition	

4. Implements appropriate follow-up care when indicated by changes in patient status including
   – documenting change in patient's medical record/progress notes
   – communicating change to patient's case manager
   – communicating change to other designated person in agency
     (i.e., assistant administrator/clinical coordinator)
   – notifying MD as appropriate	

5. Records visit on appropriate form and submits to identified person.	

(continued on next page)

Example 1-5 (continued). Competence Assessment Program Summary for Staff Providing Care to Ventilator-Dependent Patients

Attachment A

Documentation of Completion of
SNV (Intermittent Visit) Competencies

Key Behaviors	Date Met/Initials
Competency: Upon completion of orientation, the orientee will demonstrate safe practice in the home setting.	
1. Consistently uses universal precautions appropriately for home setting.	
2. Demonstrates correct agency/district specific procedure for disposal of "red bag" trash.	
3. Uses appropriate measures to ensure personal safety while in the field; includes	
4. Maintains nursing bag/supplies per agency policy and procedure.	
Competency: Upon completion of orientation, the orientee will demonstrate competence in performance of basic skills according to agency policy and procedure.	
1. Assesses patient's status using basic physical assessment skills.	

2. Performs procedures/treatments according to agency policy and procedure; may include
    a. venipuncture for routine lab draws
    b. routine wound care
    c. administration of medications
    d. blood glucose monitoring	

Competency: Upon completion of orientation, the orientee will demonstrate understanding of relationship between nurses' documentation and reimbursement.	
1. Documents need for continuing home care as appropriate on progress notes.	
2. Submits daily activity logs (Medicare patients) within 24 hours.	
3. Completes time sheet correctly and within deadlines (per policy and procedure).	
4. Notifies appropriate person if unable to make scheduled visit.	
5. Maintains effective communication with designated person in office per office/district procedures.	

Comments:

____
Employee/date

____
Supervisor/date

____
Preceptor/date

(continued on next page)

Example 1-5 (continued). Competence Assessment Program Summary for Staff
Providing Care to Ventilator-Dependent Patients

Shands HomeCare
Shands Hospital

Attachment B

Subject: **Management of Ventilator Dependent Pediatric Patients Protocol**

Policy Statement: All nurses shall complete a specialized orientation and demonstrate competency in the management of ventilator patients in the home setting **prior to being assigned to care for a home ventilator patient**.

Supporting Data: Please see Age Appropriate Protocols for general guidelines for care for pediatric patients.

Purpose: To provide guidelines for care of the ventilator dependent pediatric patient in the home setting.

Level: Interdependent; physician orders required for some interventions (*).

Issue	Interventions	Note
Admission Assessment	During the admission visit, complete the following: 1. Routine pediatric admission assessment. 2. Specific data related to patient's ventilator status: • patient's past medical history related to the vent (i.e., tolerance to vent, suctioning patterns, feeding patterns). • equipment actually in place/in use (vent type, setting, suction, oxygen, etc.). • trach (type/size/amount of air in cuff/appearance of stoma/when trach was last changed/approximate date trach due to be changed). 3. Specific plan of care in collaboration with the family.	
On-going Assessment	1. Assess & document patient's status at start of the shift and at least every 8 hours; include the following: ▶ Respiratory status (rate, breath sounds bilaterally, any independent respirations) ▶ Secretions and their characteristics ▶ Status/patency of trach ▶ Verify size of trach tube and status of cuff ▶ Heart rate and rhythm ▶ Skin color, temperature ▶ Activity level, degree of alertness ▶ Capillary refill ▶ Overall perfusion ▶ Skin integrity ▶ Bowel sounds ▶ Any complaints of pain, nausea, discomfort ▶ Last bowel movement ▶ Any edema present in dependent sites ▶ Temperature ▶ Blood pressure ▶ Pulse oximetry readings (if ordered)	Children on ventilators are more prone to GI ulcers, fluid problems, or altered cardiac output.

Age Appropriate Protocol: 10   Management of Ventilator Dependent Pediatric Patients   Copyright, 1996: Shands HomeCare

(continued on next page)

Example 1-5 (continued). Competence Assessment Program Summary for Staff Providing Care to Ventilator-Dependent Patients

Attachment B

Issue	Interventions	Note
On-going Assessment (continued)	2. Assess and document presence/status of emergency equipment; includes ▸ back-up oxygen tank if oxygen concentrator is in use ▸ back-up battery that is fully charged and ready for use ▸ portable battery-powered suction machine that is fully charged and ready for use ▸ 1 of 2 ambu bags & mask ▸ extra trach tubes (1 tube a size smaller than current tube used) & sterile water-based lubricant 3. Assess and document status of ventilator at start of shift and every 4 hours ▸ See Equipment Maintenance section for details ▸ Document on ventilator flowsheet (including humidity and oxygen)	All back-up equipment must be fully ready for immediate use (including batteries fully charged & back-up tanks full).

Prevention of Infection	1. Monitor patient for signs of infection; signs may include
	▸ Change in amount/color of secretions
	▸ Abnormal temperature
	  • Below normal temperature in infants or some neurologically impaired children
	  • Above normal temperature in children above the age of infant
	▸ Irritability
	▸ Skin color change
	▸ Diminished or abnormal breath sounds
	▸ Loss of appetite
	▸ Decrease in level of alertness
	2. Employ appropriate infection control measures to lessen risk of infection; appropriate measures include
	▸ Change vent circuits 1–2 times per week (as recommended by manufacturer).
	▸ Change water in humidifier q 24 hours
	  • Use distilled or sterile water
	  • Completely empty humidifier and refill; do not just add more water.
	▸ Clean humidifier unit every 48–72 hours (as recommended by manufacturer)
	▸ Clean suction catheters according to Infection Control policy and procedures:
	  • Rinse suction catheters after use. Catheters may be soaked in hydrogen peroxide to loosen secretions.	

Age Appropriate Protocol: 10   Management of Ventilator Dependent Pediatric Patients   Copyright, 1996: Shands HomeCare

(continued on next page)

Example 1-5 (continued). Competence Assessment Program Summary for Staff
Providing Care to Ventilator-Dependent Patients

Attachment B

Issue	Interventions	Note
Prevention of Infection (continued)	• Cleanse catheters with soap and water. Use pipe cleaners to assist with cleaning if needed. • Rinse catheters well. • Disinfect by boiling for 20 minutes or soaking in disinfectant as listed in policy for 20 minutes. • Store in clean, closed container. ▶ Clean trach tubes after changing; allow to dry & store in clean plastic bags. ▶ Clean equipment per manufacturer's or supplier's guidelines. ▶ Empty suction canisters every 8 hours and rinse out. • Change suction canisters daily. 3. Verify that caregiver/family knows how to maintain and clean all equipment. ▶ Document instruction given, caregiver/family response & return demonstration in patient's medical record.	
Equipment Maintenance	1. Evaluate and document ventilator functioning at start of shift, every 4 hours, and prn; include the following: ▶ Tidal volume ▶ Respiratory rate ▶ Peak inspiratory pressure (PIP) ▶ Inspiratory time ▶ PEEP or CPAP ▶ Humidification and temperature ▶ Mode of ventilation ▶ FiO_2 settings ▶ O_2 (analyzed) ▶ Low pressure limit ▶ High pressure limit ▶ Circuit changes 2. If pulse oximetry is used, also assess and document ▶ Oxygen sats 3. Suction equipment ▶ Verify suction pressure is in low or moderate range • Low suction setting should be used for infants. • Low to moderate setting should be used for children • High setting should NEVER be used; it can cause trauma to airway ▶ Verify that back-up suction machine is working properly.	Document on the ventilator flow sheet.

Age Appropriate Protocol: 10   Management of Ventilator Dependent Pediatric Patients   Copyright, 1996: Shands HomeCare

(continued on next page)

Example 1-5 (continued). Competence Assessment Program Summary for Staff Providing Care to Ventilator-Dependent Patients

Attachment B

Issue	Interventions	Note

Management of Equipment Failure	1. Ensure that back-up ventilator is available through DME company.
	  ▶ List DME company and emergency phone number on emergency plan.
	2. Monitor patient and ventilator for signs of equipment failure; these may include
	  ▶ Patient complaint of inadequate ventilation.
	  ▶ Persistent high or low pressure alarm states without change in the child's condition.
	  ▶ Systems failure alarm.
	  ▶ Battery will not hold charge.
	  ▶ Ventilator "sounds differently" or isn't cycling properly.
	3. If ventilator failure occurs:
	  ▶ Disconnect patient from ventilator.
	  ▶ Manually "bag" patient at same rate as ventilator settings.
	  ▶ Activate EMS if patient shows signs of deterioration while off of ventilator.
	  ▶ If spirometer is available, check expired tidal volume.
	  ▶ If oximeter is available, check oxygen saturation levels.
	  ▶ Call DME company for immediate replacement.
	  ▶ Notify MD of incident.
	4. Teach family/caregiver above measures for management of equipment failure.
	  ▶ Document instructions given, caregiver/family response & return demonstration in patient's medical record.
		Following equipment failure, the MD may wish to order tidal volume assessment.

Age Appropriate Protocol: 10   Management of Ventilator Dependent Pediatric Patients   Copyright, 1996: Shands HomeCare

(continued on next page)

Example 1-5 (continued). Competence Assessment Program Summary for Staff Providing Care to Ventilator-Dependent Patients

Attachment C

Documentation of Completion of Ventilator Competencies

Name: ____   Date: _______________________

Expected Performance/Outcome	Met	Not Met
Collaborates with physician, ventilatory vendor, and/or patient's case manager to identify appropriate outcomes of care (i.e., acceptable respiratory parameters)		
Assesses patient status at start of shift & documents in patient's medical record; assessment to include • breath sounds • respiratory rate (spontaneous/ventilator) and characteristics of spontaneous respirations (depth, effort, retractions, use of accessory muscles) • characteristics of secretions if present • skin color • capillary refill in seconds • extra trach tube at bedside (specify size)		
Assesses patient's respiratory status during the shift • when ventilator settings are changed • when patient's condition changes • before, during, and after pulmonary hygiene measures		
Identifies need for changes in ventilator settings and/or ordered treatments based on assessment of patient and knowledge of desired outcomes.		
States that ventilatory settings should be changed by ventilatory vendor whenever possible.		
States that nurses may only change ventilatory settings with direct verbal or written orders from the physician.		
Collaborates with physician about any changes in pulmonary hygiene measures.		
Performs chest PT and postural drainage per MD orders.		
Identifies need for suctioning & suctions patient using appropriate technique; includes • connecting self-inflating bag to appropriate oxygen flow source when indicated • pre- and post-oxygenating patient with self-inflating bag • using clean technique		

Copyright, 1996: Shands HomeCare

(continued on next page)

Example 1-5 (continued). Competence Assessment Program Summary for Staff Providing Care to Ventilator-Dependent Patients

Attachment C

Documentation of Completion of Ventilator Competencies

Expected Performance/Outcome	Met	Not Met
Maintains safety in home setting; includes ensuring that • no food/fluids are stored on top of ventilator • electrical cords do not drape on the floor/across walkways • self-inflating ambu bag is present • suction equipment (canister/catheter) is present • back-up portable suction is available and functional • ventilator alarms are set at correct settings and are functional • ventilator alarms are ONLY changed by ventilatory vendor with orders from MD • ventilator circuits are secured to prevent tension on the trach tube • oxygen sat monitors are at bedside when ordered • replacement trach tube is at bedside • oxygen source is available at bedside		
Implements measures to maintain safety when patient is transported outside home; includes • insuring that self-inflating bag, mask, trach kit, portable suctional equipment, and O_2 are taken with patient • insuring that ventilator alarms are turned on, placed on proper settings, and functional • reviewing with patient/caregiver that alarm settings are ONLY to be charged by the ventilatory vendor		
Assesses ventilator status at start of shift and as needed throughout shift; includes • respiratory rate (spontaneous & ventilated) • tidal volume • peak inspirator pressure • CPAP • FiO_2 • alarm limits and function • inspiratory time • humidifier level • inspired air temperature • I:E ratio • mean airway pressure • peak inspiratory flow rate • battery function and charge		

Copyright, 1996: Shands HomeCare

(continued on next page)

Example 1-5 (continued). Competence Assessment Program Summary for Staff
Providing Care to Ventilator-Dependent Patients

Attachment C

Documentation of Completion of
Ventilator Competencies

Expected Performance/Outcome	Met	Not Met
States that • the first response to an alarm situation/other perceived ventilator problem is to assess the patient for signs of respiratory distress. • if distress is present, the patient should be disconnected from the ventilator and manually bagged and airway assessed for signs of patency. • if airway is not patent, patient should be bagged or trach tube changed as indicated.		
Responds promptly to high pressure alarm states and implements appropriate assessment & intervention; includes • assesses need for suctioning, for occlusion of tube, for dislodgement of tube, & for presence of condensed water in ventilator tubing. • suctions patient if indicated • replaces trach tube if dislodged or occluded • removes water from tubing • manually bags patient and emergently notifies ventilatory vendor for high alarm states that persist despite trouble-shooting • notifies MD prn after consulting with ventilatory vendor		
Responds promptly to low pressure alarm states and implements appropriate assessment & intervention; includes • assesses for disconnects, leaks in system, or presence of "overbreathing" by patient • reconnects tubing if needed • works with patient, MD, ventilatory vendor to decrease "overbreathing" by patient • manually bags patient and emergently notifies ventilatory vendor for low pressure alarms/system leaks that persist despite trouble-shooting • notifies MD prn after consulting with ventilatory vendor		
Knows "chain of command/communication" to contact in the event a problem arises; includes • ventilatory vendor (person on call) • patient's MD • patient's case manager • assistant administrator on call		

Copyright, 1996: Shands HomeCare

(continued on next page)

Example 1-5 (continued). Competence Assessment Program Summary for Staff
Providing Care to Ventilator-Dependent Patients

Attachment C

Documentation of Completion of
Ventilator Competencies

Expected Performance/Outcome	Met	Not Met
Identifies emergency situations and intervenes appropriately. Emergency situations may include but are not limited to • trach tube dislodged • trach tube occluded • power failure • ventilator malfunction Expected interventions include • replacing trach tube • calling MD • calling ventilatory vendor • calling 911		
Performs ADL's safely; includes • turns/moves patient in bed prn without disconnecting him/her from ventilator • bathes/dresses patient prn without disconnecting him/her from ventilator and without getting water or power around trach stoma • assists patient to eat/drink; prevents spills of food/fluids around stoma • transfers patient from bed to chair, etc. prn without disconnecting him/her from ventilator		
Performs trach care per competencies outlined on trach care competency sheet.		
Establishes appropriate nonverbal communication methods with patient.		

Signatures:

____

Employee   Date

____

Preceptor/Evaluator   Date

____

Manager   Date

Copyright, 1996: Shands HomeCare

(continued on next page)

Example 1-5 (continued). Competence Assessment Program Summary for Staff Providing Care to Ventilator-Dependent Patients

Attachment D

Shands HomeCare

Summary of Joint Home Visit

Employee/Title:____ Date: ___________________

Performance Criteria	Comments	Met/Date/Initials
Patient Status Assessed		
Care Plan Revised (if needed)		
Patient Involved in Care Plan		
Care Plan Followed		
Effectiveness of Treatment Plan Evaluated		
Caring Attitude Demonstrated		
Family/S.O. Involved		
Plan for Next Visit Made		
Therapeutic Communications Skills Demonstrated		
Teaching Skills Proficient		
Concern for Health Promotion/Prevention		
Infection Control/Safety Measures Used		
Agency Procedures Followed		
Appropriate Use of Equipment Noted		

Additional Comments:

Initials/signature/title

______________________________   ______________________________

______________________________   ______________________________

Copyright, 1996: Shands HomeCare

Source: Compiled by Karen Majorowicz, SHANDS HomeCare, affiliated with SHANDS Health System, Gainesville, FL.

Example 1-6. General and Discipline-Specific Competence Assessment Policies

These checklist forms are used during both general orientation of home care staff and initial competence evaluations for medical social workers and physical therapists. The general orientation program covers the areas any patient care staff member would need to know—from home safety and infection control to methods of communication with patients. The skills checklists for specific disciplines allow the organization to identify any areas in which a staff member may require more education or training before beginning home visits.

Patient Care Staff Orientation

Employee: ____ Position: _____________________________

Orientation To:	Yes	N/A	Signature/Date
1. Basic Home Safety:			
a. Bathroom			
b. Electrical			
c. Environmental			
d. Fire			
2. Storage/Handling/Access to/Transport of Supplies			
3. Handling Medical Gases			
4. Storage/Handling/Access to/Transport of Drugs			
5. ID/Handling/Disposal of Infectious Wastes (Blood & Body Fluids/Precautions)			
6. ID/Handling/Disposal of Hazardous Waste (Cytotoxic/Chemotherapy Drugs)			
7. Infection Control			
a. Personal Hygiene (i.e., PPE & Handwashing)			
b. Aseptic Procedures			
c. Communicable Infections (TB, AIDS, etc.)			
d. Cleaning/Disinfecting Reusable Equipment			
e. Precautions to be taken (Universal Precautions, airborne transmission, direct/indirect contact, compromised immunity)			
8. Confidentiality of Pt Info			
9. Community Resources			
10. Policies/Procedures			
11. Guidelines for Appropriate Referrals, Incl. Timeliness			
12. Appropriate Action in Unsafe Situations (Staff Safety)			
13. Advanced Directives Policies/Procedures			
14. Performance of Specific Tests per Job Description			
15. Policies/Procedures Regarding Death & Dying			
16. Screening for Alleged or Suspected Victims of Abuse/Neglect Reporting			
17. Emergency Preparedness Plan & Role			

(continued on next page)

Example 1-6 (continued). General and Discipline-Specific Competence Assessment
Policies

Patient Care Staff Orientation (cont'd)

Orientation To:	Yes	N/A	Signature/Date
18. Care Coordination Based on Assessment Data & Appropriate Referrals			
19. Equipment Use/Management Relevant to Job Description			
20. Tuberculosis Program/Plan			
21. Hazardous Materials in the Workplace Program			
22. Bloodborne Pathogen Program			
23. Managing the Environment of Care: (Pt & Agency Site)			
a. Safety			
b. Fire Safety—Fire Drills, Fire Alarm System, Fire Extinguishers			
c. Security			
d. Utilities			
24. Pt Rights/Responsibilities			
25. Agency Complaint Mechanism/Medicare State Hotline #			
26. QI Program & Role			
27. On-call & Answering Service			
28. Staff Conflict-of-Interest			
29. Staff Rights Policy			
30. Interpreters/Communicating with Hearing/Speech/Visually Impaired			
31. Competency Assessment			
32. Inservices/Continuing Education (Min. Number Programs/Year)			
33. Incident/Variance Reporting Defined			
34. Management of Information:			
a. Home Care Record			
b. Computer System			
c. Library (Knowledge-based Information)			

Other: ____

____

(Note: See Job-specific Orientation Program/Checklist for Skills)

____

Employee Signature   Date

____

Supervisor Signature   Date

(continued on next page)

Example 1-6 (continued). General and Discipline-Specific Competence Assessment
Policies

Orientation Skills Checklist Medical Social Worker

Name: ____ Title: ________________________________

Skills	Competent		Comments	Date & Initial
	Yes	No		
Provide Skilled Assess of Social & Emotional Factors				
Provide Assess of Pt's Need for Long-Term Care				
Eval Home/Family Situation				
Counsel & Assist with Out-of-Home Placement				
Promote Community Services				
Provide Advocacy, Referral & Linkage with Community Services				
Counsel & Assist with Financial Problems and Entitlements				
Provide Goal-Oriented Intervention Directed Toward Management of a Terminal Illness				
Assist with Strengthening the Family Support System				
Provide Education on Community Services				
Assist with Resolution of Conflict Related to the Chronicity of Illness				
Identify & Advocate for Pts at Risk for Being Physically or Mentally Abused and/or Neglected				
Identify & Eval Pts at High Risk for Suicide				
Identify & Assist Pts with Inadequate Food and/or Medical Supplies				
Develop Care Plan According to Pt Needs				

Date of Initial Completion: _________________________________

____
Employee Signature/Title

____
Supervisor Signature/Title

(continued on next page)

Example 1-6 (continued). General and Discipline-Specific Competence Assessment
Policies

Orientation Skills Checklist Physical Therapy

Name: _______________________________________ Title: _______________________________

Skills	Competent		Comments	Date & Initial
	Yes	No		
I. Eval & Treatment of:				
1. ROM/Goniometry				
2. Strength				
3. Balance				
4. Coordination				
5. Functional Mobility				
a. Bed Mobility				
b. Transfers				
c. W/C Mobility				
d. Gait				
6. Sensation				
7. Muscle Tone				
8. Edema				
9. Endurance				
10. Positioning				
11. Home/Envir. Safety				
12. Pt/CG Teaching				
13. Body Mechanics				
II. Equipment				
1. Gait Devices				
a. Walker				
b. Crutches				
c. Hemiwalker				
d. Quad Cane				
e. Straight Cane				
f. Platforms for Walker				
g. Platform for Crutch				
2. Other				
a. Wheelchair				
b. Hoyer Lift				
c. Sliding Board				

(continued on next page)

Example 1-6 (continued). General and Discipline-Specific Competence Assessment
Policies

Orientation Skills Checklist Physical Therapy (cont'd)

Skills	Competent		Comments	Date & Initial
	Yes	No		
3. Exercise Aids				
a. Overhead Pulley				
b. Free Weights				
c. Theraband				
d. Therapotty				
e. CPM				
4. Modalities				
a. Ultrasound				
b. TENS				
c. Hot Pack				
d. Cold Pack				
e. Ice				
5. Patient Monitors				
a. Stethoscope				
b. BP Cuff				
c. Goniometer				
d. Dynamometer				
6. Splints				
a. AFO				
b. Back Brace				
c. Cervical Collar				
d. Knee Immobilizer				

Date of Initial Completion: _______________________

____
Employee Signature/Title

____
Supervisor Signature/Title

Source: Kathy J. Morgan, RNC, MPH, BSN, and Sandra L. McClain, RNC, BSH, Johnson City, TN.

Example 1-7. An Organizationwide Plan for Competence in an HME Organization

The PLATO (plan, assess, train, and orient) program used by this organization includes all aspects of the human resources function, as illustrated in the flowchart. The process begins with determining the proper qualifications for a position and then matching qualified applicants to the position. Initial evaluation or self-assessment of skills and capabilities helps the organization choose an employee, who then goes through orientation, continuing training, and ongoing competence assessment.

Due to space constraints, only a few pages of the extensive competence assessment tool are presented here.

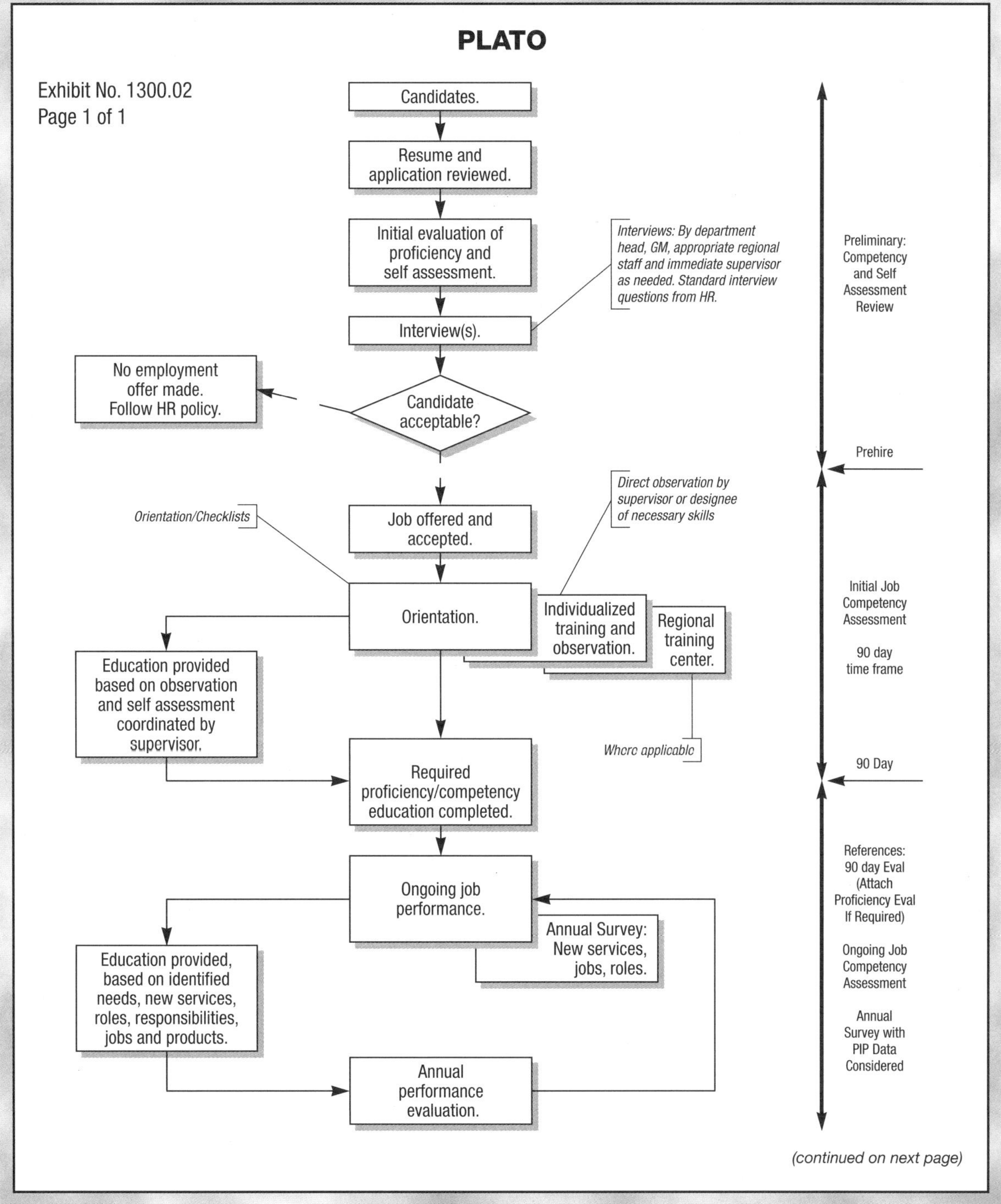

(continued on next page)

Example 1-7 (continued). An Organizationwide Plan for Competence in an HME Organization

Statement No. 1341
July 15, 1996
Supersedes 5/28/92
Page 1 of 4
Approval ________________
Approval ________________
Approval ________________

Respiratory Staff Proficiency and Education Program

Responsible

General Manager, Regional Clinical Manager, Respiratory Manager, Senior Respiratory Therapist, Staff Respiratory Therapist

Definition:

The proficiency program consists of evaluating staff knowledge and skills and providing education based on defined learning needs.

Proficiency assessment is a process for initial and continuing evaluation of the staff's ability to carry out assigned responsibilities safely, competently, and in a timely manner. The assessment evaluates whether staff capacity is equal to the requirements of the tasks assigned.

For the purpose of this policy, the proficiency program is divided into preliminary knowledge (acquired prior to employment), initial education (acquired within the first 90 days of employment), and continuing education.

Policy:

1. The competency/proficiency of all new NMC Homecare respiratory staff is assessed prior to the provision of direct patient care. Learning needs identified through the assessment are resolved.

2. The effectiveness of individualized instruction provided in response to identified learning needs of the new employee is assessed after 90 days of employment and documented on the 90-day Performance Evaluation.

3. The clinical and technical competency/proficiency of all NMC Homecare respiratory staff is assessed on a continuing basis through the Performance Improvement Program and the Clinical Operational Audit Tool (C.O.A.T.), and documented on the Annual Performance Evaluation.

4. Educational opportunities are provided to respiratory staff based on defined learning needs.

5. Full time, part time, and per diem respiratory staff are included in the proficiency assessment and education program.

6. Maintenance of staff competency/proficiency is a function of the Performance Improvement Program. A report on proficiency maintenance activities is given to the corporate office annually, in the fourth quarter report.

Procedure:

1. Assessment of *preliminary* job proficiency shall include:

   a) Verification that education and training meet the job description requirements;

   b) Appropriate evidence of current license, certification, or registration;

   c) For new respiratory therapists, verify verbally with the State Board of Respiratory Care that the therapist's license is in good standing at the time of employment, where applicable.

(continued on next page)

Example 1-7 (continued). An Organizationwide Plan for Competence in an HME Organization

Statement No. 1341 (continued)

Respiratory Staff Proficiency and Education Program

Procedure (continued):

d) For the respiratory therapist, appropriate clinical knowledge and experience for his or her assigned responsibilities as documented by successful completion of the Respiratory Competency Assessment and interview.

   i) The job candidate will complete the Respiratory Competency Assessment (exhibit 1341.01) during the interview process, prior to an offer of employment.

   ii) The interview must include discussion of the candidate's self-assessment of his or her current skill level.

2. *Initial* (90-day) education will include:

  a) Orientation to all activities in accordance with Policy Statement 1330;

  b) The new employee's direct supervisor will provide or arrange for the provision of education in response to the learning needs identified. The instruction will be completed within the first 90 days of employment.

  c) Additionally, for new supervisors assessment of proficiency will include:

   i) Understanding of the staff responsibilities associated with each level of care provided under his or her supervision as defined by policy and through orientation by the General Manager and Regional Clinical Manager;

   ii) Appropriate supervisory and, as appropriate, additional clinical knowledge and experience for his or her assigned clinical supervision responsibilities, as defined in the job description.

3. The 90-day Performance Evaluation will indicate successful completion of individualized instruction, as well as overall job performance.

4. On a *continuing* basis, competencies are measured and training provided in response to the following:

  a) Trending data from the infection control reporting system and the incident reporting system that may be related to staff education needs (Performance Improvement Committee report).

  b) Observation of clinical and technical procedures during a supervised home visit, and audit of clinical documentation (C.O.A.T. Clinical Chart audit). Supervisors will observe return demonstrations or conduct documentation audits when the following conditions exist:

   i) At least annually as part of the employee evaluation process;

   ii) When the employee is performing a new procedure or using a piece of equipment for the first time, for example:

    a) End-Tidal CO_2 Monitor.

    b) Home ventilator discharge planning and implementation.

    c) Asthma Management Program (Smart Air Ways).

    d) Antibiotic therapy administered via large-volume ultrasonic nebulizer.

   iii) The first time he or she provides care in a specialized area such as:

    a) Neonates/Pediatrics

    b) Lung transplant recipients

   iv) Whenever the employee requests it.

(continued on next page)

Example 1-7 (continued). An Organizationwide Plan for Competence in an HME Organization

Statement No. 1341 (continued)

Respiratory Staff Proficiency and Education Program

Procedure (continued):

5. Staff development needs are identified based on the assessments and questionnaires. A national survey conducted by the Department of Human Resources concerning the training and educational needs of staff will occur annually. Data related to staff proficiency are collected, aggregated, and analyzed for patterns and trends.

   a) The results of the learning needs survey are stratified by branch, region, and nationally.

   b) The results of the C.O.A.T. are stratified by branch and nationally.

   c) The Performance Improvement Program data are stratified by branch, region, and nationally.

6. Education programs, in-service programs, and educational materials (for example, journals, books, magazines, tapes) are developed, planned, or purchased based on the analysis of staff needs and trends identified. The proficiency of direct care staff members is maintained and improved through these planned educational activities.

7. Assessment of staff proficiency and subsequent training is performed when introducing new services and updated technology and/or equipment.

   a) National programs will be introduced with a staff development component included.

   b) Initiation of new programs, procedures, or equipment in a branch must be preceded by appropriate education of the staff involved. The General Manager is responsible for arranging this education.

   c) Any education provided to assure competency of staff when initiating new services or assisting staff develop new skills is documented in the employee's personnel file or on an inservice log.

8. A report about the levels of proficiency and proficiency maintenance activities is given annually in the fourth quarter Performance Improvement Committee(s) meeting minutes at the branch and national level.

(continued on next page)

Example 1-7 (continued). An Organizationwide Plan for Competence in an HME Organization

NMC Homecare

Exhibit No. 1341.0
Page 1 of 40

Respiratory Orientation Checklist and Competency Evaluation

Employee Name/Title: _______________________   Evaluator Name/Title: _______________________

Rating Scale: 1. Competent with skill/knowledge; Able to apply   2. Needs development   3. No prior experience
The NA column is used by the evaluator to indicate those areas where a self-assessment is not applicable and/or orientation will not be provided.

Phase I: General Orientation — Refer to Statement No. 1300
Completed by the General Manager or his/her designee for all respiratory employees.

Phase II: Coordination of Care
Completed by the Branch Respiratory Manager, Regional Clinical Manager, and Patient Services Manager.

	COMPLETED BY ORIENTEE					COMPLETED BY PRECEPTOR/EVALUATOR				
						Competent in Area			Re-Eval	
Skill/Knowledge	Self-Assessment (Pre-Orientation)			Last Perform Date	Orient Date	Date	Eval. Initials	Comments	Date	Eval. Initials
Job Description(s) (as applicable)										
1. Respiratory Manager	NA	1	2	3						
2. Senior Respiratory Therapist	NA	1	2	3						
3. Staff Respiratory Therapist	NA	1	2	3						
Overview of Policies and Procedures										
1. Patient Care Management System	NA	1	2	3						
2. Respiratory Care	NA	1	2	3						
3. Equipment Management	NA	1	2	3						
4. Management and Administration	NA	1	2	3						
Patient Services										
1. Morning Meeting	NA	1	2	3						
2. Referral Intake	NA	1	2	3						

(continued on next page)

Example 1-7 (continued). An Organizationwide Plan for Competence in an HME Organization

NMC Homecare

Exhibit No. 1341.0
Page 2 of 40

Respiratory Orientation Checklist and Competency Evaluation

| Skill/Knowledge | COMPLETED BY ORIENTEE | | | | | | COMPLETED BY PRECEPTOR/EVALUATOR | | | | |
| | Self-Assessment (Pre-Orientation) | | | | Last Perform Date | Orient Date | Competent in Area | | | Re-Eval | |
							Date	Eval. Initials	Comments	Date	Eval. Initials
3. Patient Acceptance "Huddle"	NA	1	2	3							
4. Admission Paperwork	NA	1	2	3							
5. Kardex	NA	1	2	3							
a. Supply Management	NA	1	2	3							
b. Patient Compliance	NA	1	2	3							
6. Key Referral Sources	NA	1	2	3							
National FT Vendor Contracts											
1. Nellcor Puritan-Bennett	NA	1	2	3							
2. Respironics	NA	1	2	3							
3. Precision Medical	NA	1	2	3							
4. Pari	NA	1	2	3							
5. Western Medical	NA	1	2	3							
6. Ceramatec	NA	1	2	3							
7. Baxter	NA	1	2	3							
8. Hudson	NA	1	2	3							
Case Management											
1. Reviewing orders for accuracy and appropriateness	NA	1	2	3							

(continued on next page)

Example 1-7 (continued). An Organizationwide Plan for Competence in an HME Organization

NMC Homecare

Exhibit No. 1341.0
Page 3 of 40

Respiratory Orientation Checklist and Competency Evaluation

Skill/Knowledge	COMPLETED BY ORIENTEE						COMPLETED BY PRECEPTOR/EVALUATOR					
	Self-Assessment (Pre-Orientation)				Last Perform Date	Orient Date	Competent in Area				Re-Eval	
							Date	Eval. Initials	Comments		Date	Eval. Initials
2. Service Classification Determination (7004)	NA	1	2	3								
3. Visit/Contact Tracking	NA	1	2	3								
4. Case Conference	NA	1	2	3								
Clinical Documentation												
1. CRS IPA/PVR	NA	1	2	3								
2. EMS IPA/PVR	NA	1	2	3								
3. Single Visit Record	NA	1	2	3								
4. Clinical Activity Pathways	NA	1	2	3								
5. Phone Contact Surveys	NA	1	2	3								
6. Clinician Notification Report	NA	1	2	3								
7. Certificate of Training	NA	1	2	3								
8. Medication Profile	NA	1	2	3								
9. Plan of Treatment	NA	1	2	3								
10. Progress Note	NA	1	2	3								
11. Clinical Service Summary	NA	1	2	3								
12. CMNs, Prescriptions, Orders	NA	1	2	3								

(continued on next page)

Example 1-7 (continued). An Organizationwide Plan for Competence in an HME Organization

NMC Homecare

Exhibit No. 1341.0
Page 4 of 40

Respiratory Orientation Checklist and Competency Evaluation

COMPLETED BY ORIENTEE						COMPLETED BY PRECEPTOR/EVALUATOR					
						Competent in Area				Re-Eval	
Skill/Knowledge	Self-Assessment (Pre-Orientation)			Last Perform Date	Orient Date	Date	Eval. Initials	Comments	Date	Eval. Initials	
13. Co-signature of documents	NA	1	2	3							
14. Assembly of the PMR (7006)	NA	1	2	3							
15. Patient Confidentiality	NA	1	2	3							
16. Security of PMRs	NA	1	2	3							
Branch Specific											
1.	NA	1	2	3							
2.	NA	1	2	3							
3.	NA	1	2	3							
4.	NA	1	2	3							
5.	NA	1	2	3							
6.	NA	1	2	3							
7.	NA	1	2	3							
8.	NA	1	2	3							
9.	NA	1	2	3							
10.	NA	1	2	3							

Source: Sharon Fowler, National Director of Respiratory Care Services, NMC HomeCare Inc., A Subsidiary of Fresenius Medical Care, North America, Lexington, MA.

Example 1-8. General and Service-Specific Orientation for Respiratory/HME Staff

The components of orientation within this competency program address both general and discipline-specific areas. Training guides and checklists are used for the necessary competencies. The supervisory visit to evaluate respiratory therapists is also part of the annual performance evaluation and occurs every six months. Although an annual evaluation is adequate, a six-month time frame shows an ongoing commitment to field evaluation of staff competence.

CHARTWELL

Employee: ___________________________

Start Date: ___________________________

New Team Member Orientation Program
Boston & Waltham Based Employees

Welcome To Chartwell:

This New Team Member Orientation Program has been developed so that you will be fully oriented to the company and prepared for new responsibilities at Chartwell. Job training will take place as prescribed by your department.

As part of this New Team Member Orientation Program, you should review all applicable items on this checklist with your supervisor. As each item is reviewed or completed, initial the space provided. When all items are completed (within 30 days), both you and your supervisor should sign the last page and forward it to Human Resources (for Home Office employees) or your HR Coordinator (Branch employees). It will be included as a required document in your personnel file.

Best wishes for an informative orientation and a successful career with Chartwell.

Phil Lockwood
Vice President, Human Resources

	Employee's Initials	Supervisor's Initials
I. New Employee Paperwork *(Urgent! Must be completed and on file by first day of employment. Employment is contingent on the completion of some of these documents. See HR on your **first day of employment**.)*		
Confidentiality Agreement	_________	_________
Employment Application	_________	_________
I-9 Employment Eligibility Verification	_________	_________
Offer Letter	_________	_________
Personal Data Form	_________	_________
W-4 Form	_________	_________
Direct Deposit Pre-notification Form *(if applicable)*	_________	_________
Driver's Insurance Information *(if applicable)*	_________	_________
Driver's License *(if applicable)*	_________	_________
Driving Record *(if applicable)*	_________	_________
Employee Health Verification *(if applicable)*	_________	_________
Non-competition Agreement *(if applicable)*	_________	_________
Professional License *(if applicable)*	_________	_________
Resume *(if available)*	_________	_________

(continued on next page)

Example 1-8 (continued). General and Service-Specific Orientation for Respiratory/ HME Staff

CHARTWELL

New Team Member Orientation Program
Boston & Waltham Based Employees

	Employee's Initials	Supervisor's Initials
II. **Benefit Orientation** – conducted by HR, every other Monday	__________	__________
III. **Introductions and Tour of Facility** *(Conducted by your supervisor. Meet your fellow team members and become familiar with the office/branch environment.)*		
Introductions to Other Team Members	__________	__________
New Employee's Work Space	__________	__________
Other Offices and Departments	__________	__________
Conference Room(s)	__________	__________
Copying/Fax/Mail Area(s)	__________	__________
Vending Machines/Cafeteria/Kitchen	__________	__________
Rest Rooms	__________	__________
Storage Areas	__________	__________
Parking	__________	__________
Other: ______________________________	__________	__________
IV. **Office and Communications Systems** *(Conducted by your supervisor. Review efficient operation of these items early on, so there will be no difficulties later.)*		
Copier	__________	__________
Fax	__________	__________
Telephones	__________	__________
Voice Mail	__________	__________
E-Mail *(if applicable)*	__________	__________
Paging Systems *(if applicable)*	__________	__________
Security/Keys *(if applicable)*	__________	__________
Other: ______________________________	__________	__________
V. **Company Information** (Discuss with your supervisor. Understand who we are, where we are going, and how we will get there.)		
History of the Company	__________	__________
Organizational Structure/Key Players	__________	__________
Mission	__________	__________
Partnership Strategy	__________	__________
Chartwell Core Values	__________	__________
Company Locations	__________	__________
Products/Services	__________	__________

(continued on next page)

Example 1-8 (continued). General and Service-Specific Orientation for Respiratory/
HME Staff

CHARTWELL

New Team Member Orientation Program
Boston & Waltham Based Employees

	Employee's Initials	Supervisor's Initials
VI. Departmental Overviews *(Attend a meeting conducted by HR approximately monthly. Discuss with your supervisor and develop an understanding of both Branch and Home Office Department operations.)*		
Professional Practice	_________	_________
Pharmacy	_________	_________
Nursing	_________	_________
NCOE Expansion	_________	_________
Materials Management	_________	_________
Field Support	_________	_________
Waltham IV & RC/HME Branch Tours	_________	_________
Planning and Marketing	_________	_________
Retail Pharmacy/Chartwell Scripts	_________	_________
Chartwell Managed Services	_________	_________
Finance/Accounting/Payroll	_________	_________
Human Resources	_________	_________
MIS	_________	_________
Reimbursement	_________	_________
VII. Employment Practices and Policies *(Supervisors and new employees should discuss these topics. Refer to Employee Handbook and/or Human Resources Policies and Procedures or call HR if you have any questions.)*		
Work Hours/Overtime Rules	_________	_________
Pay Procedures/Time Sheets/Exempt Time Off Reporting	_________	_________
Attendance Expectations	_________	_________
Paid Time Off (Vacation, Sick, Personal Days)	_________	_________
Leave of Absence (Including FMLA)	_________	_________
Expense Reports	_________	_________
Dress/Appearance	_________	_________
Professional Conduct	_________	_________
Performance Appraisal System	_________	_________
Grievance/Open Door Policy	_________	_________
Incident Reports	_________	_________
Drug Free Workplace	_________	_________
Company Property	_________	_________
No Smoking Policy	_________	_________
No Solicitation/Distribution Policy	_________	_________
Open Positions/Transfers	_________	_________
Promotions from Within	_________	_________
Employee Referral Program	_________	_________
Recognition and Length of Service Awards	_________	_________

(continued on next page)

Example 1-8 (continued). General and Service-Specific Orientation for Respiratory/ HME Staff

CHARTWELL

New Team Member Orientation Program
Boston & Waltham Based Employees

	Employee's Initials	Supervisor's Initials
VIII. Safety and Other Required Training Programs *(Home Office/Waltham employees should review these topics during the monthly General Orientation sessions.)*		
Office Safety	__________	__________
Sexual Harassment	__________	__________
Telephone Skills	__________	__________
Hazard Communications**	__________	__________
Respiratory Protection**	__________	__________
Driver Safety*	__________	__________
Bloodborne Pathogens**	__________	__________
Infection Control**	__________	__________

** For employees with direct patient contact
* For employees who drive as part of their job

	Employee's Initials	Supervisor's Initials
IX. Job Expectations *(Make sure you understand clearly your job duties and performance expectations. Discuss in depth with your supervisor now and throughout employment.)*		
Job Description	__________	__________
Performance Expectations and Standards	__________	__________
Performance Review Process/Dates	__________	__________
First Task(s)/Assignment(s)	__________	__________

(continued on next page)

Example 1-8 (continued). General and Service-Specific Orientation for Respiratory/
HME Staff

CHARTWELL Home Therapies

Interoffice Memorandum

Date: _______________________________

To: Personnel File

From: (New Team Member) _______________________________

        (Supervisor)   _______________________________

Re: **Completion of New Team Member Orientation**

Together or with HR we have completed the Chartwell New Team Member Orientation by reviewing the following items:

1) new employee paperwork;
2) introductions and tour of the facility;
3) office security and communication;
4) company history, mission, services, locations and Core Values:
5) departmental overviews;
6) employment practices;
7) safety, sexual harassment and other applicable training; and
8) job expectations.

We are satisfied that all items have been thoroughly discussed.

____
(Employee Signature)   (Date)

____
(Supervisor Signature Signature)   (Date)

(When orientation is completed and all applicable items checked off, tear off this page, sign it, and forward to the New Team Member's personnel file.)

(continued on next page)

Example 1-8 (continued). General and Service-Specific Orientation for Respiratory/HME Staff

---

CHARTWELL Home Therapies

Policy and Procedure

SUBJECT: Orientation   POLICY #: RC115
DEPARTMENT: Respiratory/HME   DATE ISSUED: 3/92
PAGE 1 OF 2   SUPERSEDES:

Policy

All new respiratory/HME employees will successfully complete a competency-based orientation prior to involvement with patients.

Procedure

The orientation is under collaborative direction of Human Resources and the new employee's immediate supervisor.

The length and scope of the orientation is dependent on the orientee's past experience and current level of knowledge and skills related to respiratory care in a home care setting. The length of the orientation period should not exceed the 90-day evaluation period.

Orientation will include, but not be limited to the following:

- Organizational policies and procedures regarding death and dying.

- Screening for abuse and neglect, appropriate to the staff member's role and responsibilities.

- Emergency preparedness.

- Other patient care responsibilities.

- Gathering of information by staff regarding the care or service provided by other members of the staff, in order to better coordinate and appropriately refer the patient.

- Types of care or service to be delivered in the patient's environment.

- Equipment management, including safe and appropriate use of equipment as applicable to care or service provided:

  - Demonstration of knowledge and competence in appropriate maintenance procedures for all equipment.

- Home safety issues, including bathroom, fire, environmental, and electrical safety.

- The storage, handling, and access to supplies, medical gases, and drugs appropriate to the care/services provided.

- The identification, handling, and disposal of infectious materials and wastes in a safe and sanitary manner and in accordance with law and regulation.

- Infection control, including: personal hygiene, precautions to be taken, aseptic procedures, communicable infections and appropriate cleaning, disinfection, and/or sterilization of equipment and supplies.

- Confidentiality of patient information.

- Appropriate policies and procedures.

- Community resources as applicable to the care or service provided.

(continued on next page)

Example 1-8 (continued). General and Service-Specific Orientation for Respiratory/ HME Staff

CHARTWELL Home Therapies

Policy and Procedure

SUBJECT: Orientation
PAGE 2 OF 2

- Guidelines for appropriate referrals, including timeliness.

- Appropriate action in unsafe situations.

- Any specific tests to be performed by the staff.

- The organization's policies and procedures regarding advance directives.

Each employee is responsible for the completion of all required orientation documentation.

Completed orientation documentation will be returned to Human Resources.

All orientation documentation will be kept in the employee's personnel file.

Orientation to new therapies, equipment techniques, etc., will be provided prior to use.

Review of the respiratory care practitioner's competency will be evaluated by formal review and supervised home visits quarterly.

A patient services representative's performance will be reviewed by the operations supervisor on an ongoing basis and will be evaluated by a formal review process annually.

Approved: ____

Reviewed: ____

Revised: ____

(continued on next page)

Example 1-8 (continued). General and Service-Specific Orientation for Respiratory/ HME Staff

---

CHARTWELL Home Therapies

Policy and Procedure

SUBJECT: Training Guide and Checklist

DEPARTMENT: Respiratory/HME

PAGE 1 OF 1

POLICY #: RC116

DATE ISSUED: 7/94

SUPERSEDES: 3/93

Policy

Each Patient Service Representative and Respiratory Care Practitioner will be trained in the techniques listed on the attached "Training Guide and Checklist."

Procedure

When training and compliance has been completed, the Training Guide and Checklist will be maintained in the respective personnel folders, located in the Human Resources Department. For items not applicable, the letters "NA" will be placed in the appropriate space.

Approved: ____

Reviewed: ____

Revised: ____

(continued on next page)

Example 1-8 (continued). General and Service-Specific Orientation for Respiratory/
HME Staff

Name: _______________________________

Training Guide and Checklist

ORIENTATION	Date of Instruction	Demonstration	Comments	Trained By
Company Background				
Company Goals				
Customer Service				
Image: Self & Company				
Work Rules				
Admissions, Qualifications, and Insurance Verification				
The Referral Process				
Out-of-Service Referrals				
Coverage Criteria Guidelines				
A Mock Referral				
Vehicle				
DOT/FDA Regulations (RCPs/PSRs)				
Inventory Levels (RCPs/PSRs)				
Loading/Unloading (PSRs)				
Maintenance/Cleaning (PSRs)				
Padding & Restraints (PSRs)				
Safety Procedures (PSRs)				
Theft Prevention (RCPs/PSRs)				
Paperwork				
Accident Reporting				
Admission Assessment				
Advanced Medical Directive				
Apnea Monitor Log Sheet				
Client Files				
Communication Log				
Consent for Service				
Consult Sheets				
CPAP Certificate				
CPAP Outcome Measurement				
Current Pick Up Reports				
Current Rental Reports				
Daily Order Log (PSRs)				

(continued on next page)

Example 1-8 (continued). General and Service-Specific Orientation for Respiratory/ HME Staff

Training Guide and Checklist

ORIENTATION	Date of Instruction	Demonstration	Comments	Trained By
Paperwork (continued)				
Discharge Summary				
Equipment Checklist				
Equipment Repair Forms				
Expense Reports				
Field Service Tickets				
General Complaint Log				
Home Safety Checklist				
Incident Reports				
Inventory Control (PSRs)				
Notification Letter (Green Half-Sheet/Instructions)				
Open Order Reports				
O_2 Daily Calibration Log				
Plan of Care				
Plan of Treatment				
Pneumogram Log Sheet				
Manometer Verification Log				
Productivity Reports				
Progress Note				
Purchase Order Requisition				
Rights and Responsibilities				
Route Sheets				
Time Sheets				
Trach/Sxn Supply List				
Vehicle Manifest (PSRs)				
Work Order Slip				
Disaster Plan				
Product Knowledge				
Infection Control/Cleaning				

Oxygen
  Gaseous Cylinders/Regulators
  Concentrators
    Devilbiss
      MC44-90				

(continued on next page)

Example 1-8 (continued). General and Service-Specific Orientation for Respiratory/ HME Staff

Training Guide and Checklist

ORIENTATION	Date of Instruction	Demonstration	Comments	Trained By
Disaster Plan				
Product Knowledge (continued)				

Oxygen (continued)
  Concentrators
    Devilbiss
      MC4490DS
      MC84DS
    Puritan Bennett
      Companion 590
  Liquid Cylinders
  Liquid Portables
    1000
    550
    500				

Suction
  Gomco
    Gastric
    Stationary
  Devilbiss (Portable)
  Schucco (Stationary)				

Resuscibaby/ResusciAnnie/ Chris Clean				
Respirometer				
Manual Resuscitator				

End-Tidal CO_2 Monitors
  Novametrlx
  Biochem				

Oximeter
  Nellcor
  LifeCare
  Ohmeda				

Heaters/Humidifiers
  Conchatherm
  Conchatherm III
  Cascade
  Fisher Paykel
    HC100
    MR 480				

(continued on next page)

Example 1-8 (continued). General and Service-Specific Orientation for Respiratory/ HME Staff

Training Guide and Checklist

ORIENTATION	Date of Instruction	Demonstration	Comments	Trained By
Disaster Plan				
Product Knowledge (continued)				
Heaters/Humidifiers (continued)				
Ohmeda Bottom Heater				
Puritan Bennett Stick Heater				
Phototherapy				
Wallaby I				
Wallaby II				
Joey				
Ohmeda				
Peak Flow Meter				
Micro Spirometer				
BIPAP				
Quantum Bilevel Vent				
CPAP				
Healthdyne				
Tranquility				
Quest				
LifeCare				
CP-100				
Respironics				
Aria				
Sleep Easy III				
Remstar				
Remstar Choice				
CPAP Supplies				
Adams Circuit				
Monarch Mini Mask				
Respironics Mask				
Sullivan Mask				
Healthdyne				
Respironics Humidifier				
Nebulizer (Pulmo-Aide)				
PariJet				
Pulmo-Aide Traveler				
Devilbiss Ultrasonic Portable				
Ultra Neb 99				

(continued on next page)

Example 1-8 (continued). General and Service-Specific Orientation for Respiratory/
HME Staff

Training Guide and Checklist

ORIENTATION	Date of Instruction	Demonstration	Comments	Trained By
Disaster Plan				
Product Knowledge (continued)				
Mist Tent Ohmeda				
Compressor				
O_2 Bleed-in Procedures				

Apnea Monitor
   Healthdyne
   970S
   900
   Modules
   Modem
   Aequitron
   9500				

2 Channel Pneumogram Multichannel Pneumogram Downloading at MGH				

Ventilator
   Cargo Battery System
   Puritan Bennett 2801
   Aequitron LP6
     LP6 Plus
     LP10
   LifeCare PLV-100
      PLV-102
      Thompson Ventilator
   Puritan Bennett
     Maxivent				

IPPB Puritan Bennett				
ThAIRapy Vest				
TBMask Fitting				

I have been instructed on all policies and procedures relating to the above.

____

Signature   Date

____

Printed Name of the Above Signature

(continued on next page)

Example 1-8 (continued). General and Service-Specific Orientation for Respiratory/ HME Staff

Chartwell Home Therapies
Training Guidelines

Office Safety

Purpose

The purpose of this training program is to create an awareness, and educate and inform employees about the potential dangers in the work environment and to provide guidelines for correcting conditions which frequently lead to accidents and injuries.

Who Should Attend and How Often

All new employees to the company should attend this Office Safety Training Program within 30 days of their hire date. This training is part of the New Team Member Orientation. Employees are required to attend this program only at time of hire.

Who Delivers This Training and How It Is Delivered

In each branch, HR Coordinators are responsible for delivering this program to new employees as they come on board. At the corporate office, the HR department will deliver the program monthly as part of the regular orientation program. Participants will be verbally introduced to the importance and objectives of this topic. The trainer will then show a video and administer a post-test.

Program Objectives

At the completion of this program employees should be able to:

1. Identify the principle safety hazards in the work place.

2. Describe how upturned carpet edges, slippery floors and floor conditions can pose a safety hazard in the office.

3. Explain the importance of good housekeeping in maintaining a safe office environment.

4. Explain the safety hazard caused by chairs, file cabinets and other furniture left in corridors and other heavy traffic areas.

5. Demonstrate proper lifting techniques for moving heavy loads in the office.

6. Identify the location of fire extinguishers and fire exits and know the proper evacuation procedures.

Required Materials

1. Video "Office Safety: It's A Jungle In There" (20 minutes)

2. Office Safety Post-Test and Post-Test Answer Key

3. In-Service Attendance Record

Record Keeping

1. Trainers should provide post-test, grade it upon completion, give one copy to the employee and keep one copy for the personnel file.

2. The In-Service Attendance Record should be kept by the HR Coordinator (field) or HR staff (corp).

(continued on next page)

Example 1-8 (continued). General and Service-Specific Orientation for Respiratory/
HME Staff

Chartwell Home Therapies
Training Guidelines

Office Safety

Program Content

I. Office Safety Hazards

a. Tripping Hazards—the # 1 cause of accidents

   1. Causes

      Carpet edges

      Extension cords

      Cluttered floors

   2. Solutions

b. Clothing on the Job

   1. Dangers of loose fitting clothing

   2. Importance of proper footwear.

c. Slipping Hazards

   1. Wet tile/marble floor surfaces

   2. Track rugs and boot baskets

d. Running Accidents

   1. Running through offices

   2. Racing up or down stairs

   3. Stairway access doors

e. Dangers in Food Areas

   1. Slippery floors near coffee machines

   2. Burns

   3. Overload electrical shocks

f. Dangers in Not Using Office Furniture Correctly

   1. Using desk tops to reach high places

   2. Using desk chairs as step ladders

   3. Overloading file cabinets

g. Lifting Hazards

II. Fire Hazards in the Office

a. Causes of Office Fires

   1. Overloaded circuits

   2. Lit cigarette butts

b. Training Employees for Fire Hazard Awareness

   1. Fire alarm system location

   2. Fire exit locations

   3. Fire extinguisher location and use

(continued on next page)

Example 1-8 (continued). General and Service-Specific Orientation for Respiratory/ HME Staff

CHARTWELL

Office Safety Program—Post-Test

Employee Name: ____ Date: ______________________

The above named employee has been oriented to basic office safety. This post test should be graded immediately following completion of the training. A copy is provided to the employee and a copy should be provided to the personnel file as documentation of attendance.

Post Test

T   F   1. Only female office workers need to be aware of catching their clothing in office equipment.

T   F   2. Unsecured extension cords are a frequent cause of falls in the office.

T   F   3. Wet boots or overshoes should be left by your desk.

T   F   4. File/desk drawers should be kept closed when they're not being used.

T   F   5. A desk top may be used as substitute ladder in order to reach something on an overhead shelf as long as the desk surface is free of a slipping hazard.

T   F   6. Heavy material can be stored anywhere in a filing cabinet where there is room.

T   F   7. Heavy materials should be lifted with knees bent.

T   F   8. Counter surfaces around refreshment areas should be kept clean and dry.

T   F   9. After sounding the fire alarm, you should gather your personal belongings and hurry out of the office.

T   F   10. Material may be stored on the floor near a desk if it is well marked and obvious to everyone in the immediate area.

T   F   11. Running on stairs is only permitted in an emergency.

T   F   12. Employees only need to know the emergency exit routes before a fire starts.

T   F   13. Falls are the leading cause of accidents in the office.

T   F   14. Sharp edges are the only hazard associated with a desk.

T   F   15. New employees are more prone to accidents in some cases.

Employee Signature ____

Source: Chartwell Home Therapies, Waltham, MA.

Example 1-9. Orientation Checklist to Guide Competence Assessment of Home Health Nurses

This checklist divides topics for initial training into logical sections and includes some seemingly trivial, yet important, issues, such as using mailboxes and the phone system. Field observations with a preceptor are also included. This form does not establish competence, but rather, documents that certain activities have been completed. A checklist dedicated to competence could be developed based on this one.

Orientation Checklist
Registered Nurse

Employee Name: _______________________________ Date of Employment: _______________

	Initials	Date
Agency Introduction	__________	__________

- Introduction to Staff Members
- Agency Layout
- Phone System
- Mailboxes

Agency Information _________ _________

- Philosophy, Principles, and Objectives
- Organizational Chart
- Scope of Services/Role of Other Disciplines
- Patient Confidentiality and Responsibility/Patient Bill of Rights

Personnel Policies _________ _________

- Name Badge
- Completion of Required Agency Forms for Employment: Personnel File Checklist
- Employee Manual: – Probation
  – Evaluations
  – Grievance Procedures
  – Benefits
  – Payroll Policies
- Hepatitis B Vaccine
- Job Description

Daily Routine Responsibilities _________ _________

- Case Management/Staff Assignments
- Weekly Schedules/Scheduling of Visits
- On Call Procedure: Call Back Book
- Per Diem Staff: Procedure For Daily Assignments
- Day Sheets/Organization of Visits
- Payroll/Mileage Tabulation/Time Cards

(continued on next page)

Example 1-9 (continued). Orientation Checklist to Guide Competence Assessment of Home Health Nurses

Orientation Checklist
Registered Nurse

Daily Routine Responsibilities (continued)   Initials   Date

- Beeper Use
- Communication Techniques/Call In Schedule
- Paperwork Turn In
- Lab Deliveries
- Nursing Bag Contents and Policy
- Bag and Handwashing Technique

Policy and Procedure Manual Review

- Manuals
- Emergency Procedures
- Accidents/Incidents: Occurrence Report
- Blood and Body Fluid Precautions/Infection Control
- Safety Orientation and Training

Medicare Review

- Explanation of Home Health Care Guides and Reimbursement

Paperwork Review

- Patient Chart and Divisions
- Paperwork Flow: – Referral and Treatment Care Plan
  - 485, 486, 487
  - Interim Orders
  - Socioeconomic Sheet
  - Patient Care Plan
  - Skilled Nursing Visit Report
  - Case Conference/Progress Notes
  - Clinical Notes
  - Lab Results Flow Sheet
  - Discharge Summary
  - Post-Hospitalization Plan of Treatment Updates
  - Transfer Summary
  - Initial Visit Documentation: Initial Visit Packet
  - Guidelines for Patient Evaluation/Initial Assessment and Ongoing Process

(continued on next page)

Example 1-9 (continued). Orientation Checklist to Guide Competence Assessment of Home Health Nurses

Orientation Checklist
Registered Nurse

Supervision of Patient Care   Initials   Date

- Review of Home Health Aide Job Description
- Home Health Aide Care Plan
- Home Health Aide Visit Report
- Home Health Aide Supervisory Visit

Agency and Community Resources

- Contact Services
- DME Ordering and Use in Home
- Staff Meetings
- Inservice Requirements

Medisense Operation and Maintenance

Quality Assurance

- Clinical Record Reviews

Field Experience

- Observation Visits with Designated Preceptor/Observation of Physical Assessment
- Patient Visit with Preceptor Observing/Performance of Physical Assessment
- Caseload Arrangement/Patient Visits

____

Signature of Employee   Date

____

Signature of Person(s)   Date

____

Responsible for Orientation   Date

Example 1-10. Determining Frequency of Assessment for Bereavement Counselors

The following table illustrates how a hospice organization—after identifying the qualifications and competencies needed for bereavement counselors—might decide which of the competencies should be reviewed annually by prioritizing each competency in terms of its relationship to family volume, risk, and potential difficulty.

Example:

Hospice

Staff Position: Bereavement Counselor

Paper Qualifications for Hire:

- Application
- 2 references
- Documented interview
- Evidence of M. Div. or equivalent experience
- Driver's license
- I-9 Form
- Resume
- Job description
- etc.

Competencies/Skills	Low Volume	High Risk	Problem Prone	Assess During Orientation	Assess Annually
Bereavement Assessment			X	X	
Spiritual Assessment			X	X	
Identify Family Needs			X	X	
Develop Bereavement Plans of Care			X	X	X
Counseling			X	X	X
Communication			X	X	X
Coordination of Services			X	X	X

Section 2: Assessing Individual Competence

This section presents various tools from home health, hospice, home medical equipment, and pharmacy organizations. They vary in specificity according to employees' job responsibilities and levels of proficiency. Most of the tools and forms can be adapted to fit service- and organization-specific requirements (for example, cost-effectiveness, ease of use).

Example 2-1. Case Study for Assessment of Clinical Competence

A case study is one way to demonstrate competence for a specific job category. Case studies can be tailored to individual patient populations and competence levels, and can be changed as needed. They can also be used to customize existing assessment programs to include job-specific competencies, and they are excellent for assessing clinical knowledge.

Assessment of Clinical Competency
Infectious Disease Module

Employee: ____ Date: _____________________

Successful completion and review of the following topics:

________ identifying an appropriate antibiotic, including route, dose and duration, for a given diagnosis or culture result

________ knowledge of potential side effects of antibiotics, antifungals, antivirals

________ knowledge of recommended infusion times and type of IV line

________ Cockroft and Gault equation to estimate a patient's renal function

________ knowledge of optimum times to draw aminoglycoside and vancomycin serum levels

________ evaluating daily dose of an antibiotic, antifungal, antiviral in a patient with compromised renal function and/or liver function

Employee's signature: _______________________________________ Date: _____________________

Manager's signature: _______________________________________ Date: _____________________

Employee has demonstrated competency in the above areas by case observation/training.

Trainer/Observer Pharmacist: _______________________________ Date: _____________________

Note: Please give this form to your manager for file.

(continued on next page)

Example 2-1 (continued). Case Study for Assessment of Clinical Competence

Infectious Disease Module

Name: ____   Date: ___________________

Answer the following questions using the given materials

Case A: OP is a 35-year-old woman who has complained of anorexia, weight loss, and fever for the past 2 months. Her past medical history is significant for an aortic aneurysm with insufficiency that resulted in an aortic valve replacement (porcine) three years prior to admission. She had dental work 3 months prior to admission. Her WBC = 14,000/mm3 with a slight left shift: all other laboratory results were within normal limits. She is not on any medications currently and does not have any allergies. She was diagnosed with bacterial endocarditis. Later four of four cultures grew gram positive cocci growing in clusters, which was later identified as *Staphylococcus aureus*.

Question 1: What antibiotic(s) would be a good empiric choice for this diagnosis (circle all)?
1. cefazolin
2. vancomycin
3. ciprofloxacin
4. penicillin and gentamicin
5. rifampin
6. amphotericin B

Question 2: If the culture grew *enterococcus faecalis*, what would be a good drug regimen (circle all)?
1. cefazolin
2. vancomycin
3. ciprofloxacin
4. penicillin and gentamicin
5. rifampin
6. amphotericin B

Question 3: If the culture grew methicillin-resistant *staphylococcus aureus* (MRSA), how would OP's therapy differ?

Question 4: If vancomycin was prescribed, what are some of the drug related problems or toxicities that may be encountered (circle all):
1. hepatotoxicity
2. "red man syndrome"
3. renal toxicity
4. ototoxicity
5. metallic taste

Question 5: When are ideal times for drawing vancomycin peak and trough serum levels?

Question 6: Why is the combination of a penicillin with an aminoglycoside recommended for *enterococcus faecalis*?

(continued on next page)

Example 2-1 (continued). Case Study for Assessment of Clinical Competence

Infectious Disease Module

Question 7: How is creatinine clearance calculated? Where are some sources to look up the formula?

Question 8: Which antibiotics need to be adjusted for renal function (circle all)?
1. trimethoprim/sulfamethoxazole
2. pentamidine
3. amphotericin B
4. ciprofloxacin
5. penicillin

Question 9: For the following blood culture and sensitivity result, what would be the best choice of drug (excluding cost):

ciprofloxacin	< = 1	S	
gentamicin	8.0	I	
tobramycin	2.0	S	
piperacillin	>64	R	*Pseudomonas aeruginosa*
timeth/sulf	>2/38	R	
ceftazidime	>16	R	
imipenem	< = 4	S	Answer: ______________
aztreonam	>16	R	
amp/sulbactam	>16/8	R	

Case B: AP is a 55-year-old-male who recently suffered a severe fracture of his left distal tibia, which required surgical intervention for open reduction of the fracture. His course was stable following surgery; however, 2 weeks postoperatively, AP developed pain and swelling in his left calf. His symptoms worsened and he now presents with increasing local tenderness, warmth, swelling and erythema. AP is afebrile and has the following laboratory results:

WBC = 7,800/mm3
ESR = 80 mm/hr
serum creatinine = 0.9 mg/dl
BUN = 12.5 mg/dl

Osteomyelitis was diagnosed based on the above and x-ray findings.

Question 1: If the bone tissue culture grew *E. Coli* and ceftixozime is ordered, what is the dose, interval and infusion rate?

Question 2: If gentamicin is ordered, what are the ideal peak and trough levels in mcg/ml?

Question 3: If the culture grows out *Pseudomonas aeruginosa*, can ciprofloxacin be used? If so, what dose, route and duration?

(continued on next page)

Example 2-1 (continued). Case Study for Assessment of Clinical Competence

Infectious Disease Module

Question 4: If AP was 8 years old, how would the dose of ciprofloxacin be adjusted?

Question 5: If AP was diabetic, how might his disease state affect antibiotic therapy (circle all)?
1. less tissue penetration
2. higher serum levels
3. more toxicity
4. poor glucose control
5. need higher doses

Case C: AT is an 11-year-old girl s/p heart transplant diagnosed with mucormycosis from an aortic aneurysm sensitive to amphotericin. She has a Broviac line in place and parents were taught how to infuse amphotericin for a duration of 8 weeks then every other day for 6 months. Serum creatinine is 0.7 mcg/ml. She is on multiple medication including oral magnesium and potassium supplements.

Question 1: What are some of the toxicities that can be encountered with this medication (circle all)?
1. hepatoxicity
2. "red man syndrome"
3. renal toxicity
4. ototoxicity
5. metallic taste
6. chills and rigors

Question 2: What laboratories should be routinely checked to monitor toxicity (circle all)?
1. serum creatinine
2. electrolytes
3. liver function tests
4. serum amphotericin levels
5. blood sugar

Example 2-2. High-Tech, Population-Specific Competence Evaluations for Private Duty Nurses

Registered nurses and licensed practical nurses at this high-tech pediatric organization are assessed at the time of application, annually thereafter, and whenever new skills or equipment are introduced. Assessment during the initial interview is a way to ensure not only that nurses are competent in the necessary areas but that they are aware of the needs of the patient population. This also gives the organization an opportunity to educate the applicant in procedures specific to Pediatric Special Care. The forms cover general competencies, such as infection control and documentation, as well as clinical procedures. They can be used for observation and to record documented evidence of competence, such as a written exam for tracheostomy care.

Pediatric Special Care, Inc.

Applicant Skills Competency Evaluation

Applicant Name: ________________________________ Date: ____________________

City of Residence: ______________________________ Preferred Shifts: ______________

Skills Demonstration

Verbalized (V)   Actual Demonstration (A)   No Experience (N)   Unacceptable Demonstration (U)

Trach	G-tube	NGT	NMT
assmt ___________	assmt ___________	measurement ________	med adm __________
care ___________	care ___________	insertion ___________	equip prep__________
change ___________	feeding ___________	placement__________	
tie change___________	change ___________	**Vent**	**Broviac**
suctioning __________		LP 6 ______________	drsg ______________
		LP 10 _____________	flush _____________
		BiPAP _____________	med adm __________
		hospital____________	

Additional in-service needed on:

Trach____

Gastrostomy ____

Nasogastric ____

NMT ____

Vent/BiPAP____

Broviac ____

Interviewer's Signature____

Copy to: Staffing Coordinator ____________ Clinical Nurse Manager ____________ President ____________

(continued on next page)

Example 2-2 (continued). High-Tech, Population-Specific Competence Evaluations for Private Duty Nurses

Pediatric Special Care, Inc.

RN Skills Competency Evaluation

☐ Applicant ☐ Annual ☐ New skill/equipment

Name: _______________________________________ Date of Review: _______________________

	No Experience	Demonstrated	Competent		
			Y	N	I
Nursing Process					
1. Plan of Treatment					
a. Conducts health history/physical exam					
b. Develops a problem list					
c. Reviews POT prior to providing care					
d. Establishes and revises goals					
e. Provides services according to POT					
f. Conducts initial assessment, vital signs, and developmental assessment					
g. Recognizes discriminating observations in patient's changing condition					
h. Coordinates care with parents, clinical manager, physician, & other team members					
2. Documentation					
a. Writing is legible, neat					
b. Problems noted in margins					
c. Documents initial assessments & developmental level					
d. Assesses and documents patient's response to treatment					
e. Completes and signs notes, time sheets, etc., in a timely manner					
3. Infection Control					
a. Washes hands prior to patient contact					
b. Wears gloves, gowns, masks, goggles when appropriate					
c. Properly disposes of used needles. Does not recap needles					
d. Utilizes Universal Precautions					
e. Demonstrates proper disinfection techniques with equipment					
Clinical Skills					
1. Gastrostomy					
a. Assessment of stoma site					
b. Care of stoma site					

(continued on next page)

Example 2-2 (continued). High-Tech, Population-Specific Competence Evaluations for Private Duty Nurses

Pediatric Special Care, Inc.

RN Skills Competency Evaluation

	No Experience	Demonstrated	Competent		
			Y	N	I
Clinical Skills (continued)					
1. Gastrostomy (continued)					
c. Administration of gastrostomy feedings					
d. Removal and insertion of G-tube					
2. Nasogastric					
a. Measurement of NGT					
b. Insertion of NGT					
c. Placement check of NGT					
d. Administration of NGT feedings					
3. Nebulizer Mist Therapy					
a. Preparation of equipment					
b. Medication administration					
4. Apnea Monitoring					
a. Purpose of procedure					
b. Turns on and off monitor					
c. Position of pads and belt					
d. Low heart rate alarm intervention					
e. Apnea alarm intervention					
f. Loose lead alarm intervention					
5. Tracheostomy					
a. Assessment of stoma site					
b. Care of stoma site					
c. Tracheal suctioning					
d. Trach tie change					
e. Trach change					
6. Ventilator Management					
a. Low pressure alarm					
b. High pressure alarm					
c. Routine ventilator care					
d. Ventilator circuit and humidifier change					
e. Backup power source					

(continued on next page)

Example 2-2 (continued). High-Tech, Population-Specific Competence Evaluations for Private Duty Nurses

Pediatric Special Care, Inc.

RN Skills Competency Evaluation

	No Experience	Demonstrated	Competent		
			Y	N	I
Clinical Skills (continued)					
7. Broviac					
a. Dressing change					
b. Heparinization of catheter					
c. Injection cap change					
d. Blood withdrawal					
e. Medication administration					
f. Complications and emergency care					
8. PICC Line					
a. Assessment of site and dressing change					
b. Heparinization of catheter					
c. Blood withdrawal					
d. Complications and emergency care (migration)					

Comments:

Additional in-service needed on: ____

Signature of Evaluator ____ Date _______________

(continued on next page)

Example 2-2 (continued). High-Tech, Population-Specific Competence Evaluations for Private Duty Nurses

Pediatric Special Care, Inc.

LPN Skills Competency Evaluation

☐ Applicant ☐ Annual ☐ New skill/equipment

Name: _______________________________ Date of Review: _______________________________

	No Experience	Demonstrated	Competent		
			Y	N	I
Nursing Process					
1. Plan of Treatment					
a. Able to assist in developing a problem list					
b. Reviews POT prior to providing care					
c. Provides services according to POT					
d. Conducts initial assessment, vital signs, and developmental assessment					
e. Coordinates care with clinical manager, physician, parents & other team members					
f. Coordinates changes to clinical manager, physician, parents & other team members					
2. Documentation					
a. Writing is legible, neat					
b. Problems noted in margins					
c. Documents initial assessments & developmental level					
d. Assesses and documents patient's response to treatment					
e. Completes and signs notes, time sheets, etc., in a timely manner					
3. Infection Control					
a. Washes hands prior to patient contact					
b. Wears gloves, gowns, masks, goggles when appropriate					
c. Properly disposes of used needles. Does not recap needles					
d. Utilizes Universal Precautions					
e. Demonstrates proper disinfection techniques with equipment					
Clinical Skills					
1. Gastrostomy					
a. Assessment of stoma site					
b. Care of stoma site					
c. Administration of gastrostomy feedings					
d. Removal and insertion of G-Tube					

(continued on next page)

Example 2-2 (continued). High-Tech, Population-Specific Competence Evaluations for Private Duty Nurses

Pediatric Special Care, Inc.

LPN Skills Competency Evaluation

	No Experience	Demonstrated	Competent		
			Y	N	I
Clinical Skills (continued)					
2. Nasogastric					
a. Measurement of NGT					
b. Insertion of NGT					
c. Placement check of NGT					
d. Administration of NGT feedings					
3. Nebulizer Mist Therapy					
a. Preparation of equipment					
b. Medication administration					
4. Apnea Monitoring					
a. Purpose of procedure					
b. Turns on and off monitor					
c. Position of pads and belt					
d. Low heart rate alarm intervention					
e. Apnea alarm intervention					
f. Loose lead alarm intervention					
5. Tracheostomy					
a. Assessment of stoma site					
b. Care of stoma site					
c. Tracheal suctioning					
d. Trach tie change					
e. Trach change					
6. Ventilator Management					
a. Low pressure alarm					
b. High pressure alarm					
c. Routine ventilator care					
d. Ventilator circuit and humidifier change					
e. Backup power source					
7. Broviac					
a. Dressing change					
b. Heparinization of catheter					

(continued on next page)

Example 2-2 (continued). High-Tech, Population-Specific Competence Evaluations for Private Duty Nurses

Pediatric Special Care, Inc.

LPN Skills Competency Evaluation

	No Experience	Demonstrated	Competent		
			Y	N	I
Clinical Skills (continued)					
7. Broviac (continued)					
c. Injection cap change					
d. Blood withdrawal					
e. Medication administration					
f. Complications and emergency care					
8. PICC Line					
a. Assessment of site and dressing change					
b. Heparinization of catheter					
c. Blood withdrawal					
d. Complications and emergency care (migration)					

Comments:

Additional in-service needed on: ____

Signature of Evaluator ____ Date _______________________

(continued on next page)

Example 2-2 (continued). High-Tech, Population-Specific Competence Evaluations for Private Duty Nurses

Trach Competency Exam

(For multiple choice questions, select the best answer)

Name: ____ Date: _______________

1. What is the normal respiratory rate for a newborn?
    A. 30–40 breaths/minute
    B. 120–160 breaths/minute
    C. 40–60 breaths/minute
    D. 80–100 breaths/minute

2. What do you look for when evaluating respirations?
    A. color, rate, alertness
    B. sounds, rhythm, quality, rate
    C. sound, secretions
    D. rate, rhythm

3. One reason for a tracheostomy is:
    A. a diagnosis of BPD
    B. to prevent respiratory infection
    C. to provide direct access for secretion removal
    D. severe respiratory distress

4. Name some signs which indicate trach care must be done more often:

5. Is Vaseline a good lubricant for a trach change?

6. Which of the following would describe the proper fit of a child's trach tie?
    A. a finger cannot be placed under the tie
    B. three fingers can be placed under the tie
    C. one finger can be placed under the tie

7. The correct length to insert the suction catheter into the trach during suctioning is to:
    A. insert the catheter to one inch below the tip of the trach
    B. insert the catheter until resistance is met
    C. insert the catheter to just below the tip of the trach

8. List (2) indications that suctioning is needed:
    1.
    2.

9. What are (3) signs of a lack of oxygen?
    1.
    2.
    3.

(continued on next page)

Example 2-2 (continued). High-Tech, Population-Specific Competence Evaluations for
Private Duty Nurses

Trach Competency Exam

10. Why should you carry a trach tube one size smaller than the one in use?

11. List (3) causes for an apnea monitor to alarm:
    1.
    2.
    3.

12. What is the first thing you do when you hear an apnea monitor alarming?

13. When might CPT be helpful?

14. A respiratory treatment should be interrupted or discontinued before it's completed when:
    A. the child falls asleep
    B. the child's respiratory distress has resolved
    C. the child indicates he/she no longer wants the treatment
    D. observable untoward reactions are noted, such as an increased pulse rate, and/or respiratory distress

15. The length of time an oxygen tank will last depends on _______________ and _______________.

Source: Pediatric Special Care, Inc, Troy, MI.

Example 2-3. Competency Checklist for New Employees in a Pharmacy

Upon completion of orientation, new pharmacists' competencies are assessed in the areas covered in this form. As illustrated in this excerpt, the form includes all areas within the company with which the new pharmacist may need to interact to successfully perform his or her job. The original list is very complete, consisting of 26 total categories and covering job requirements, company philosophy, and structure.

CHARTWELL Home Therapies

New Pharmacist Orientation Checklist

Name: _______________________________________ Date of Hire: _______________________

Branch: _______________________________________ Supervisor: _______________________

Training Topic	Preceptor's Initials	Date
1. Complete "General Orientation" Checklist for New Hires	_________	_________
2. Overview of Pharmacy Operations Department:		
• Role and Objectives	_________	_________
• Scope of Services	_________	_________
• Organization and Management	_________	_________
• Team Approach (RPh, PSC, etc.)	_________	_________
• Owner Hospitals	_________	_________
• Joint Ventures/Clinics	_________	_________
3. Review of Job Descriptions & Responsibilities:		
• Qualifications	_________	_________
• Position Relationships	_________	_________
4. Overview of Pharmacy Service Delivery System:		
• Referral/Admissions Process	_________	_________
• Patient Information Sheet	_________	_________
• Pharmaceutical Care	_________	_________
• Operations Flow	_________	_________
• Distribution Process	_________	_________
5. Service Categories:		
• Full Service	_________	_________
• Co-Management	_________	_________
• Pharmacy Services Only	_________	_________
6. Communication:		
• Nursing/Pharmacy Meetings	_________	_________
• Liaison Nurses	_________	_________
• Change of Status	_________	_________
• Conference Calls	_________	_________
• Memos	_________	_________
• Branch Board Meetings	_________	_________
• Patient Boards	_________	_________
• Scheduling	_________	_________

(continued on next page)

Example 2-3 (continued). Competency Checklist for New Employees in a Pharmacy

CHARTWELL Home Therapies

New Pharmacist Orientation Checklist

Training Topic	Preceptor's Initials	Date
7. Insurance Verification:		
• Initial Insurance Clearance and Approval	_________	_________
• Follow-Up on Changes in Therapy (Managed Care)	_________	_________
• Re-Authorization Periods for Managed Care	_________	_________
• Payor Specific Guidelines for Therapy Types	_________	_________
• Patient Information/Physician Change Forms	_________	_________
8. Materials Management:		
• Overview of System	_________	_________
• Introduction to Maxim	_________	_________
• Purchasing/Ordering	_________	_________
• Receiving	_________	_________
• Accounts Payable	_________	_________
• Inventory Control:	_________	_________
– HHCA Numbers	_________	_________
– Kit Codes	_________	_________
– Inventory vs. Non-Inventory Items	_________	_________
– Physical Inventory	_________	_________
– Inventory Transfers	_________	_________
– Inventory Requests	_________	_________
– Contracts	_________	_________
– PDL	_________	_________
– MDL	_________	_________
• Controlled Substances:	_________	_________
– Purchasing	_________	_________
– Receiving	_________	_________
9. Receiving/Documenting Prescriptions & Order Changes:		
• Overview	_________	_________
• Patient Clinical Records - Confidentiality	_________	_________
• Prescriptions/Prescription Files	_________	_________
• Obtaining Physician's Orders	_________	_________
• Follow-Up Calls to MD for Continuing/Stopping Therapy	_________	_________
• Calls to MD to Recommend Changes in Therapy	_________	_________
• Calls to VNA's for Labs, Clinical Updates, Reporting Changes in Orders	_________	_________
• Communication with Chartwell Nurse (VMX, Paging)	_________	_________
• Calls to Patients - Dosage Changes	_________	_________
• Communication Notes, Note Format	_________	_________
• Change of Status	_________	_________

(continued on next page)

Example 2-3 (continued). Competency Checklist for New Employees in a Pharmacy

CHARTWELL Home Therapies

New Pharmacist Orientation Checklist

Training Topic	Preceptor's Initials	Date

9. Receiving/Documenting Prescriptions & Order Changes: (continued)
- Generic Prescription:
  - Therapy Types
  - Initial Generic Script
  - Changes in Generic Script
  - Billing Codes
  - HHCA Codes
  - Script Log Number
  - Enter & Print Generic Script in Computer System
- Ancillary Prescription
- Batch (Compounding) Records
- Laboratory Results
- Change in Prescription or Usage
- Creation of Medication Profile, Documenting Changes
- Medispan Patient Drug Information Sheets
- Pick Slip
- Controlled Substances

10. Clinical Pharmacy:
- Attend Documentation Section of New Clinician Workshop
- Attend RPh Tocolytic Therapy Training Program (if providing Maternal-Fetal Health Services)
- Plans of Treatment
- Obtaining and Interpretation of Discharge/Physician Orders
- Appropriateness of Therapy, Dosages, Allergy
- Drug Stability/Compatibility
- Dosage Calculations
- Laboratory Work, Interpretation, Retrieval, Transcription onto Flow Sheet, Trending
- First Dose and Anaphylaxis Order
- Flushing Protocols
- Delivery Schedules
- Follow-Up Calls
- Communication to Nursing
- Patient Charting, Note Format, Documenting Conversations on Patient Care
- Attending Physicians
- Clinical Follow-Up Regarding Drug Related Problems, Outcomes

(continued on next page)

Example 2-3 (continued). Competency Checklist for New Employees in a Pharmacy

CHARTWELL Home Therapies

New Pharmacist Orientation Checklist

Training Topic	Preceptor's Initials	Date

10. Clinical Pharmacy (continued):
- Communication/Dissemination of Information
- Patient Status Change Form
- Re-Hospitalized Patient File

11. Pharmaceutical Care:
- Review of JCAHO Standards
- Initial Pharmacy Assessments
- Medication Care Plans
- Retrieve Patient Data
- Clinical Recommendations
- Identify Problems/Outcomes
- Develop Pharmaceutical Monitoring Plan
- Medication Profiles: Initial, Revisions, Medispan Patient Drug Information Sheets
- Laboratory Results, Monitoring

12. Pharmacy/Operations Computer System:
- Overview of System
- Log-In Procedures
- Access Code
- Drug-Linking
- Generic Prescriptions
- Order Entry
- Compounded Prescriptions:
    - Generating Batch Record - New Prescription
    - Verification of Batch Record Information
    - RPh Initials
    - Drug, Dosage, Number of Doses
    - Route, Vehicle, Container, Volume, Overfill, Frequency, Quantity
    - Infusion Rate
    - Mix/End Date
    - Inventory Selection
- Prescription Labels
- Expiration Date
- SIG/Instructions
- Altered Compounding Instructions
- Compounded vs. Home Mix

(continued on next page)

Example 2-3 (continued). Competency Checklist for New Employees in a Pharmacy

CHARTWELL Home Therapies

New Pharmacist Orientation Checklist

Training Topic	Preceptor's Initials	Date

12. Pharmacy/Operations Computer System (continued):
- Stat/ASAP/Today
- Free Drug
- Prescription Refills:
  - Dosage Change
  - Refill Same Quantity
- Voiding a Prescription
- MAR
- Doctor's Letters
- Prescription Numbering
- Prescription Labels
- Lot Numbers
- Therapy Codes
- Delivery Codes/Reasons
- Expiration Dates
- Printing

13. Operations:
- System Log-In
- Billing Codes
- Prescription Log
- Ship Order Log
- Copies
- Procedure
- Line Numbers
- Printing
- Picking and Checking
- Ship Order Verification:
  - Matching Paperwork
  - Purpose/Process
  - Errors in Verification
  - Pump/Pole Billing
  - Credit Memos
  - Printing
- Patient Supplies
- Change in Prescription
- Change in Usage
- Generic Prescription

Source: Scott Reid, Pharm D, Chartwell Home Therapies, Waltham, MA.

Example 2-4. Written Tests for Competence Evaluation of Therapists and Rehabilitation Staff

A committee composed of management and field staff developed these and other written tests for competence evaluation. Questions are credited to the staff person who wrote them so they will not be administered to him or her. Creating these tools resulted in several advantages to the organization:

- Staff involvement sparked some informative discussions about competence and gave them a sense of pride in their unique contributions;

- The tests were integrated with existing assessment systems whenever possible to avoid creating parallel, redundant systems (such as mandatory in-services, additional interviews at the time of hire); and

- The information gained from the tests was used to further develop the competence program.

In addition to the examples shown, there are specific tests for new equipment, special skills (such as PICC line placement), and mandatory services (such as safety); a checklist used during covisits with a supervisor or professional colleague; and a home health aide competence program.

VNA & Hospice of Pomona/San Bernardino

Agency Specific Questions for
Rehab Staff Competency

Name of employee taking test: ____
           Last   First

1. All VNA staff should wash their hands both before and after contact with each patient.

    True   or   False

2. Blood and body fluids are the contaminants that necessitate protective wear in Universal Precautions.

    True   or   False

3. VNA staff do not need to request the patient's permission before using the telephone in their home if the call is made for VNA business use only.

    True   or   False

4. Confidentiality of patient information is a subjective issue. If the VNA staff believe that certain individuals need to know confidential information, then the VNA allows this information to be disclosed.

    True   or   False

____
Signature   Date

(continued on next page)

Example 2-4 (continued). Written Tests for Competence Evaluation of Therapists and Rehabilitation Staff

VNA & Hospice of Pomona/San Bernardino

Speech Therapy Competency Questions

Name of speech therapist taking test: ____

                                Last   First

1. What would you include in an assessment or eval for a CVA or swallowing client?

2. If you had a referral for a disorder that was unfamiliar to you (e.g., lung cancer, laryngectomy), what resources would you use to obtain information on that disorder?

Answers to Speech Therapy Questions

Question 1 Response

CVA: I would use a test battery such as the Boston Diagnostic Aphasia Examination. This is a comprehensive test which can evaluate all areas of communication, e.g., speech, auditory comprehension, naming, reading, and writing, etc. Voice and pragmatics, i.e., social use of language, are judged clinically throughout the evaluation.

Question 2 Response

I would consult books and references within my own professional library. If I didn't have an appropriate reference available, I would go to my local university library. I'd also confer with my colleagues. Speech Pathology is a profession whereby one is always going to be confronted with an unfamiliar disorder. However, certain practices are always going to be used. The American Cancer Society has a great deal of material available for professionals which gives thorough background information from which treatment and support strategies may be employed.

(continued on next page)

Example 2-4 (continued). Written Tests for Competence Evaluation of Therapists and Rehabilitation Staff

---

VNA & Hospice of Pomona/San Bernardino

Occupational Therapy Questions

Name of occupational therapist taking test: _______________________________________

Last   First

1. What are the precautions a patient should follow after a total hip replacement?

2. What is standard adaptive equipment that a patient with a total hip replacement needs?

3. What is the OT's role in providing care for a patient with COPD? (Chronic obstructive pulomary disease)

Signature ____   Date _______________

Answers to Occupational Therapy Questions

1. A. Do not flex your hips more than a 90° angle.
   B. Do not allow your leg to internally rotate.
   C. Do not cross your ankles or legs.

2. A. Dressing stick   E. Commode chair or raised toilet seat
   B. Reacher   F. Shower chair
   C. Sock aid   G. Shower hose
   D. Long handled sponge

3. The OT should educate the patient in regards to proper breathing patterns as well as techniques regarding energy saving and pacing for self care and ADL. Treatment might also include upper extremity exercise program to increase endurance and activity.

(continued on next page)

Example 2-4 (continued). Written Tests for Competence Evaluation of Therapists and Rehabilitation Staff

VNA & Hospice of Pomona/San Bernardino

Physical Therapy Competency Questions

Name of therapist taking test: ____

                                     Last   First

1. What are some contraindications to ultrasound?

____

____

____

____

____

____

____

2. Describe 2 parameters for use of CPM.

____

____

____

____

____

____

____

3. Match ultrasound parameters for:

Heating:	$.5w/cm^2$ x 5' pulsed 20%
Tendon healing:	$.15-.25\ w/cm^2$ x 15' pulsed 20%
Bone healing:	$.5w/cm^2$ x 5' pulsed 20%
Phonophoresis:	$1-2w/cm^2$ x 5-10' continuous

____

Signature of PT   Date

(continued on next page)

Example 2-4 (continued). Written Tests for Competence Evaluation of Therapists and Rehabilitation Staff

VNA & Hospice of Pomona/San Bernardino

Answers to Physical Therapy Questions

1. Possible answers:

    Pregnancy

    Pacemaker

    Not over eyes

    CA

    Not directly over central nervous system

    Not over gonads

2. Possible answers:

    Set protective ROM according to MD orders

    Duration 8–24 hours (according to diagnosis)

    TKR usually 6–8 hours daily—can be broken up into segments (example 2 hr on 2 hr off, etc.)

    For comfort—can be used with ice.

    Used first three weeks after surgery.

3. Answers for US parameters:

    Heating: $1\text{-}2w/cm^2$ x 5-10' continuous

    Tendon healing: $.5w/cm^2$ x 5' pulsed 20%

    Bone healing: $.15\text{-}.25\ w/cm^2$ x 15' pulsed 20%

    Phonophoresis: $.5w/cm^2$ x 5' pulsed 20%

(continued on next page)

Example 2-4 (continued). Written Tests for Competence Evaluation of Therapists and Rehabilitation Staff

---

Visiting Nurse Association of Pomona/San Bernardino

Annual RN Competency Exam—Test #1

Name: ____ Date: ____________ Score: ____________
     Last   First

MULTIPLE CHOICE - Circle the best answer.

1. Before giving the adult patient his prescribed daily dose of Digoxin, the nurse finds the patient's apical pulse is 54. Before administering the drug the nurse should:
   A. Re-check the original order, then give the dose
   B. Hold the medication and notify the physician
   C. Break the tablet in half and give the patient half the dose
   D. Give the medication in divided doses over the next 3 hours

2. Components of Universal Precautions would include all of the following *except:*
   A. Wearing goggles to perform daily bath
   B. Wearing gloves to start a peripheral IV
   C. Wearing gloves and gown to clean up a patient with bloody diarrhea
   D. Disposing of used syringes without recapping needles

3. Toxic effects of many chemotherapeutic drugs is/are:
   A. Bone marrow depression
   B. Nausea/vomiting
   C. Alopecia
   D. A and B only
   E. All of the above

4. Your bedridden patient has developed a right lower lobe pneumonia. She is on oral antibiotics for the infection. Which of the following nursing interventions is not appropriate?
   A. Perform percussion and postural drainage every four hours
   B. Auscultate breath sounds every 2–4 hours
   C. Administer expectorants as ordered
   D. Encourage low fluid intake to prevent fluid overload

5. There is a small grease fire in the kitchen. You would do all of the following *except:*
   A. Move your patient out of the home
   B. Call "911"
   C. Pour water on the flames
   D. Use baking soda or a kitchen fire extinguisher if the fire is small and well contained

6. Your elderly patient tells you that her son is physically abusive to her. You notice bruises on her wrists and arms. All of the following actions are appropriate *except:*
   A. Notify your supervisor
   B. Confront the son with this information
   C. Work with your supervisor to notify the physician, protective services and social worker if appropriate
   D. Wait to see if the incident happens again
   E. B & D

(continued on next page)

Example 2-4 (continued). Written Tests for Competence Evaluation of Therapists and Rehabilitation Staff

Visiting Nurse Association of Pomona/San Bernardino

Annual RN Competency Exam—Test #1

7. Your COPD patient is on 2 LPM O_2 via nasal prongs. She complains of anxiety and feeling "air hungry". Which of the following interventions is not appropriate:

   A. Increase oxygen to 10 LPM

   B. Elevate HOB to 90°

   C. Assist patient to perform "pulse-lipped" breathing

   D. Administer ordered IPPB treatment

8. Clozaril is a psychotrophic drug used in the treatment of refractory schizophrenia. Which laboratory values must be closely monitored?

   A. BUN and Creatinine

   B. CBC with differential

   C. Serum iron and iron binding capacity

   D. Serum glucose

9. A Stage III dermal ulcer is characterized by all of the following *except:*

   A. Full thickness tissue loss

   B. May be covered by eschar

   C. May have undermining sinus tract formation

   D. Painful wound base

10. Your patient's peripheral IV has been in for 24 hours. Which of the following does *not* indicate a need to restart this IV?

    A. Blanching, edema at site

    B. Reddened. painful at site

    C. Positive blood return

    D. Obstructed flow

11. The physician has calculated that the patient should receive 2500 ml of intravenous fluid every 24 hours. The IV administration set delivers 15 gtts/per milliliter.

    The flow rate should be: Utilize this formula: $\dfrac{\text{Volume infused} \times \text{gtts/cl}}{\text{total time in min}}$

    A. 20gtts/min

    B. 24gtts/min

    C. 26gtts/min

    D. 27gtts/min

12. The CADD PCA can be used for:

    A. Continuous delivery of medication

    B. Patient activated doses without a continuous infusion

    C. Continuous delivery of medication with patient activated doses

    D. All of the above

(continued on next page)

Example 2-4 (continued). Written Tests for Competence Evaluation of Therapists and Rehabilitation Staff

Visiting Nurse Association of Pomona/San Bernardino

Annual RN Competency Exam—Test #1

13. Children with Cystic Fibrosis have characteristic stools that are:

    A. Watery and green

    B. Large, clay colored and frothy

    C. Tarry and frequent in number

    D. Loose white and odorless

14. Medication order is Phenobarb elixir 3mg. Stock in the patient's home is 15mg/5cc. What dose should you give?

    A. 1.0cc

    B. 1.5cc

    C. 0.5cc

    D. 0.25cc

15. When assessing a patient's lung sounds the nurse should:

    A. Only be concerned with listening at the front of the chest below the clavicles

    B. Auscultate at the apex and bases posteriorly by asking the patient to inhale & exhale deeply

    C. Have the patient cough to clear the upper airway passages: it isn't necessary to auscultate with a stethoscope

16. Veraparmil is a commonly used medication used mainly for the treatment of:

    A. Arthritis

    B. Hay fever

    C. Atrial arrhythmias

    D. Gastric ulcer

17. A client with a diagnosis of bronchogenic carcinoma would not be considered for the hospice program because:

    A. The physician will not commit to a 6 month or less life expectancy

    B. He does not have adequate caregiver

    C. He refuses to sign the DNR form

    D. All of the above

18. A subcutaneous injection of Heparin is preferably administered into which of these sites:

    A. The deltoid muscle

    B. The abdomen

    C. The anterior thigh

    D. The gluteus maximus

19. A DLS include all of the following *except:*

    A. Bathing and dressing

    B. Toileting

    C. Feeding

    D. Reading the newspaper

(continued on next page)

Example 2-4 (continued). Written Tests for Competence Evaluation of Therapists and Rehabilitation Staff

Visiting Nurse Association of Pomona/San Bernardino

Annual RN Competency Exam—Test #1

20. You are caring for a comatose patient. All medications are given via the nasogastric tube. You notice the wife pouring medication directly from the bottle into the NG tube. As part of your family education you would:
    A. Explain to the wife to always check tube for placement first, otherwise she is doing fine
    B. Explain that you must check tube placement and measure the correct dosage of medication every time
    C. Explain that you must measure the correct medication dosage, but there is no need to check tube placement because you did that this morning
    D. Ignore the situation as she is obviously doing her best in a difficult situation

21. Mrs. White is receiving 40 units Regular Insulin at 7:30 am daily. On the basis of this, you know that the most likely time for her to experience an insulin reaction is:
    A. By 8:00 am
    B. At 4:00 pm
    C. During the night
    D. Around 11:00 am

22. The HIV virus is spread via all of the following *except:*
    A. Hugging and kissing on the cheek
    B. Sex—vaginal, oral or anal
    C. Through receiving blood transfusions or blood clotting factors or transplants infected with the virus
    D. Sharing diabetic insulin needles
    E. A & B

23. A common side effect of codeine is:
    A. Diarrhea
    B. Constipation
    C. Slurred speech

24. Tetracyclines are potent broad spectrum antibiotics which:
    A. Cause discoloration of the teeth
    B. Are phototoxic
    C. Are inactivated by antacids
    D. All statements are true

25. Which of the following may be classified as a narcotic analgesic with antitussive effect?
    A. Demerol
    B. Meperidine
    C. Morphine
    D. Codeine

Are there any nursing procedures you need inservicing on?

☐ No　　☐ Yes (Specify)____

Questions for this test were compiled from the CAHSAH (California Association for Health Services at Home) Staff Assessment Tool and the Visiting Nurse Association of American Procedure Manual.

(continued on next page)

Example 2-4 (continued). Written Tests for Competence Evaluation of Therapists and Rehabilitation Staff

Visiting Nurse Association of Pomona/San Bernardino

Annual RN/LVN Competency Exam—Test #1

Name: ____ Date: ____________ Score: ____________

Last   First

Test Answers

1. B	14. A
2. A	15. B
3. E	16. C
4. D	17. D
5. C	18. B
6. E	19. D
7. A	20. B
8. B	21. D
9. D	22. A
10. C	23. B
11. C	24. D
12. D	25. D
13. B	

Guide for Scoring for RN

-1 .... 96%

-2 .... 92%

-3 .... 88%

-4 .... 84%

-5 .... 80%

-6 .... Fail

Guide for Scoring for LVN

-1 .... 95%

-2 .... 90%

-3 .... 85%

-4 .... 80%

-5 .... Fail

Source: Karen Green, President, and Marsha Fox, Vice President, VNA & Hospice of Southern California.

Example 2-5. Technical Competence Assessment for Pharmacy

Although it only addresses one aspect of a pharmacy technician's job, this is a good tool for assessing aseptic technique while mixing sterile product (a specific job requirement) and may be adapted to assess other staff members as well. Criteria are well defined and the observer has space to note specific comments and to identify problems. Similar tools can be developed to cover each competency of a job.

Panorama City Inpatient Pharmacy

Pharmacy Technician Competency Assessment

Date:____

Pharmacy Technician:_________________________________

Evaluating Pharmacist: _______________________________

Each activity is graded   S = Satisfactory   U = Unsatisfactory

	Grade (S/U)	Action
1. Proper attire (shoe cover, head covers, and gowns).		
2. Proper handwashing with povidone-iodine or chlorhexidine scrub for one minute upon entering area and for 15 seconds on re-entry.		
3. All work performed at least 6 inches inside the LFH or on the non-perforated surface inside the BCH.		
4. No disruption of sterile airflow.		
5. Proper needle and syringe manipulation:		
A. removal of syringe from package and proper handling		
B. removal of needle from package and proper handling		
C. attachment of needle to syringe.		
6. Transfer of drugs		
A. ampoules to intravenous solutions (i.e., changing needle to filter needle)		
B. addition of drug to IV solution		
C. addition of dissolved drug to IV solution.		
7. Proper swabbing technique.		
8. Visual inspection of final product.		

Additional Comments:

Corrective Actions:

(continued on next page)

Example 2-5 (continued). Technical Competence Assessment for Pharmacy

Panorama City Inpatient Pharmacy

Pharmacist Competency Assessment

Antibiotic Monitoring	Met	Not Met	Action
1. Demonstrates knowledge of the department's Antibiotic Monitoring Protocols (Policy 1501.0 and 1501.1).			
2. Estimates the creatinine clearance using serum creatinine and patient data.			
3. Estimates the LBW and adjusted body weight in obese patients.			
4. Demonstrates knowledge of clinical factors, use of diuretics, and disease states which affect serum creatinine (e.g., dehydration, ESRD, CF).			
5. Understands assumptions made in using any of the pharmacokinetic models for estimating antibiotic doses, and recognizes those clinical situations where the answers generated are inaccurate.			
6. Adjusts dose of an antibiotic based on renal or hepatic function, depending on the primary route of elimination.			
7. Determines if the prescribed antibiotic therapy is appropriate/necessary.			
8. Validates appropriateness of the aminoglycoside dose ordered by the physician.			
9. Calculates appropriate aminoglycoside dose for Gentamicin, Tobramycin & Amikacin (both single daily dosing and multiple daily dosing).			
10. For aminoglycoside therapy, calculates Kel, Cmin, and dosing interval based on the patient's random levels.			
11. Determines appropriate vancomycin dose based upon patient's weight, age, renal function and disease state.			
12. Selects appropriate times for random or trough levels and interprets/evaluates lab data.			
13. Demonstrates knowledge of common diagnostic procedures ordered for patients as they relate to antibiotic use.			
14. Demonstrates knowledge of common laboratory values and normal ranges as they relate to antibiotic use and disease states.			
15. Validates appropriateness of antibiotic dosing for pediatric patients.			
16. Demonstrates knowledge of drug costs associated with antibiotic therapy, and recommends cost effective alternatives when appropriate.			

(continued on next page)

Example 2-5 (continued). Technical Competence Assessment for Pharmacy

Panorama City Inpatient Pharmacy

Pharmacist Competency Assessment

Antibiotic Monitoring	Met	Not Met	Action
17. Demonstrates knowledge of the common infectious disease states and the most likely microbial etiologic causes including but not limited to the following: Sepsis AIDS Pyelonephritis Intrabdominal infections Pelvic infections Sexually transmitted diseases FUO in immunocompromised patients Endocarditis Osteomyelltis Meningitis Upper and lower respiratory tract (Pneumonia, otitis media, bronchitis) Cellulitis Diabetic foot infections Urinary tract infections			
18. Understands the various pharmacological & pharmacokinetic characteristics of the antimicrobials used, including all cephalosporins, Primaxin, Aztreonam, Amphotericin B, Bactrim, Pentamidine, Gancyclovir DDC, Fluconazole, Aminoglycosides, Vancomycin, Itraconazole, Extended spectrum penicillins, Foscarnet, Clindamycin and Metronidazole.			
19. Demonstrates familiarity with antimicrobial literature and ability to locate drug information as required.			

Date:____

Pharmacist: ____

Evaluation ID Physician: ______________________________

(continued on next page)

Example 2-5 (continued). Technical Competence Assessment for Pharmacy

Panorama City Inpatient Pharmacy

Pharmacist Competency Assessment

TPN Monitoring	Met	Not Met	Action
1. Demonstrates knowledge of the TPN Protocol (Policy 1201.0 & 1201.1).			
2. Identifies clinical disease states for which TPN therapy is appropriate.			
3. Familiar with the organization's standardized TPN formulations.			
4. Calculates daily IV caloric count, based on TPN, Intralipid and other Dextrose containing IV solutions administered.			
5. Identifies signs and symptoms of fluid overload.			
6. Recommends electrolyte/insulin and other adjustments for TPN, as required.			
7. Can identify signs of infection in a patient receiving TPN therapy.			
8. Proficient in utilizing the LMS/RMS data systems to retrieve patient information and laboratory data.			
9. Effectively communicates with physicians and recommends appropriate therapy adjustments, based on hospital guidelines and protocols.			
10. Coordinates patient care effectively with medical staff, nursing staff, and laboratory personnel.			
11. Completes all appropriate documentation per hospital/pharmacy policies, procedures, and protocols.			

Date:____

Pharmacist: ____

Evaluator: ____

Source: Howard Kramer, RPh, and W. Weinstein, MD.

Example 2-6. Competence Assessment for Patient Education Regarding Equipment

The following forms are used as a guide for evaluating care staff who teach patients about the use and care of apnea monitors, enteral pumps, and oxygen concentrators. The evaluation for each piece of equipment covers the basic steps that must be covered (including pre-setup expectations, procedures to be covered, and documentation to be completed after the education session). The evaluation allows for differences in individual teaching styles, but all components must be included.

Name ____

Apnea Monitor Set-up
(usually taught at hospital)

(Steps need not necessarily be done in the order listed.
Each person will have his/her own style of teaching, but each step must be included sometime during the visit.)

	Yes	No
Pre set-up:		
selects monitor that has been checked out and is patient ready	________	________
gathers appropriate paperwork and supplies (2 sets of everything except cable)	________	________
verifies hospital room # and time of teach	________	________
carries appropriate ID as applicable	________	________
Washes hands prior to set-up	________	________
Teaches parents/caregivers and requests return demo as appropriate:		
Preparation of home and baby's room:	________	________
place on sturdy table	________	________
secure all electrical wires	________	________
clipboard, event sheet, pen flashlight near monitor	________	________
Function and features of monitor:		
charging light	________	________
on/off switch: location and function	________	________
loose lead light/alarm: location and function	________	________
apnea time delay set at prescribed level	________	________
apnea light/alarm: location and function	________	________
bradycardia alarm set at prescribed level	________	________
bradycardia alarm/light: location and function	________	________
tachycardia alarm set at prescribed level	________	________
tachycardia alarm/light: location and function	________	________
alarm reset button: location and function	________	________
memory light/alarm: location and function	________	________
Use of accessories:		
preparation of skin and electrodes for good contact	________	________
placement of belt and electrode pads	________	________
lead wire intact (loop test)	________	________
carrying case: how to use (do not *leave* monitor in case)	________	________

(continued on next page)

Example 2-6 (continued). Competence Assessment for Patient Education Regarding Equipment

Apnea Monitor Set-up

	Yes	No
General Care of Monitor:		
review of general cleaning procedures	_________	_________
monitor check-out procedure (return demo)	_________	_________
review of event sheet	_________	_________
battery charging procedures	_________	_________
Emergency Procedures:		
all emergency numbers at monitor and each phone	_________	_________
CPR instructed by hospital personnel prior to discharge	_________	_________

Completes appropriate paperwork:

	Yes	No
AO#, SN, supplies included on delivery receipt	_________	_________
monitor checklist completed	_________	_________
any problems noted on initial plan of care	_________	_________
initial assessment begun (continue on first home visit)	_________	_________
apnea monitor release of liability signed by parents/caregivers	_________	_________
informs parents/caregivers of routine and after-hours call procedure	_________	_________
stresses to re-order supplies before critically low	_________	_________
CPR poster given	_________	_________
parents/caregivers given and briefly explained:		
Rights and responsibilities document	_________	_________
Safety pamphlet #3	_________	_________
Satisfaction questionnaire	_________	_________
Events sheets supplied	_________	_________
FDA safety alert	_________	_________
Catalog or Airway brochure	_________	_________
Cleaning instructions	_________	_________
Apnea monitor booklet	_________	_________

Competency verified by: _________________________________ Date: _______________

Comments: ____

____

____

(continued on next page)

Example 2-6 (continued). Competence Assessment for Patient Education Regarding Equipment

Name____

Enteral Pump Set-up

	Yes	No
Selects appropriate equipment and supplies:		
Enteral pump with battery fully charged	_________	_________
IV pole	_________	_________
Pump sets: 30 days' supply	_________	_________
formula: 30 days' supply	_________	_________
paperwork and instruction manual	_________	_________
Washes hands prior to set-up	_________	_________
Instructs patient/caregiver and requests return demo, as appropriate:		
fill pump set with formula (water may be used for initial instruct)	_________	_________
hang set on IV pole and prime tubing	_________	_________
plug power cord in properly grounded outlet	_________	_________
press key labeled "on" to activate power	_________	_________
set desired rate in ml/hr by pressing (or)	_________	_________
with clamp closed, thread properly primed tubing and drip chamber into drip chamber guide and thread latex tubing around rotor	_________	_________
connect to NG, J-tube, G-tube, etc.	_________	_________
open roller clamp	_________	_________
press run/start/hold button to initiate feeding	_________	_________
Additional pump features:		
in order to change delivery rate, pump must be put on "hold" mode (rotor not turning)	_________	_________
vol limit feature may be used to preset amount to be delivered	_________	_________
vol delivered feature is a check of how much has been delivered since last reset (for simplicity, may advise caregiver to ignore these 2 features)	_________	_________
"off" button will turn pump off—it will also "wipe out" visual display of vol fed/delivered	_________	_________
Kangaroo 224 allows for settings in 5cc increments only. (The K-324 allows for 1cc increment settings.)	_________	_________

(continued on next page)

Example 2-6 (continued). Competence Assessment for Patient Education Regarding Equipment

---

Enteral Pump Set-up

	Yes	No

Additional tips:

    always irrigate tube if feeding interrupted for more than 5 minutes

    try not to hang formula more than 4 hours at a time during day, 6–8 hours at night

    always start feeding with formula at room temperature; very cold formula will cause cramping

Review cleaning instructions with patient/caregiver:

use bag for 24 hours, then discard

always unplug pump prior to cleaning it

wipe over casing with damp cloth; do not use detergents or alcohol

clean whenever spillage occurs (when formula hardens it is very difficult to remove)

clean drop sensor with Q-tip dampened with warm water

wipe pump rotor with damp cloth and Q-tip
(rotors must be clean for accurate rate delivery)

use caution when cleaning near electrical receptacle on back

Completes appropriate paperwork:

AO#, SN recorded on delivery receipt

delivery checklist completed, home safety documented

rights, responsibilities document given

satisfaction questionnaire left

home safety pamphlet #3 given

Airway brochure/catalog given

instruction manual provided

Competency verified by: ____ Date: ______________

Comments: ____

____

____

(continued on next page)

Example 2-6 (continued). Competence Assessment for Patient Education Regarding Equipment

---

Name____

Oxygen Client Initial Assessment

	Yes	No
Washes hands prior to patient visit	________	________
Assesses patient/caregivers' knowledge of equipment use and maintenance. Reviews as necessary:	________	________
proper liter flow and hours of use	________	________
filter cleaning	________	________
placement of concentrator (for proper circulation)	________	________
turning on and setting flow both on primary and back-up system	________	________
alarm situations	________	________
cannula and tubing change frequency; cleaning humidifier, if applicable	________	________
use of water-based vs petroleum-based lubricants	________	________
re-ordering of supplies before critically low	________	________
frequency of therapist/technician visits	________	________
Assesses homecare environment; makes suggestions as appropriate:		
fire safety (exit routes, smoke detectors, fire extinguishers)	________	________
hazards in home (discussed and documented)	________	________
appropriate storage of portable cylinders	________	________
no-smoking signs posted (patient's choice; check for availability of signs)	________	________
Assesses support system and psychosocial status:		
able and willing caregiver available, if needed	________	________
appropriate family support	________	________
Checks equipment:		
analyzes concentrator, checks flow	________	________
checks electrical cord for proper condition/use	________	________
checks back-up tank (pressure in tank, tank support and position)	________	________
checks for appropriate supplies	________	________
Documents above on assessment form	________	________
Documents problems on care plan	________	________

Competency verified by: ___________________________________ Date: ________________

Comments: ____

____

____

Source: Laurie Piersma, RN, RRT, Airway Oxygen Inc, Grand Rapids, MI.

Example 2-7. Medical Competence Exam for Hospice Physicians

The Visiting Nurses Association of Western Pennsylvania uses this exam as a competence evaluation for the physicians who care for hospice patients. The medical director sends the question to each physician, who answers it and returns the form to the organization. The physician's response is recorded and a copy of the correct answer, as well as the calculations used and other information on the use of morphine for hospice patients, is returned to him or her.

Name ____   Date _____________________

Hospice Medical Competency Examination

Task: To convert *oral morphine* dose to *IV morphine.*

Problem: Mrs. Windsor is a 60-year-old patient with intractable pain from metastatic bone disease. She is currently using 210 mg. of MS Contin q 12 hours routinely with 60 mg MSIR ordered q 4 hours PRN for breakthrough pain. She has used 8 doses of MSIR in the past 24 hours. Despite her current medication regimen she describes her pain as constant and rates it at an "8" on a scale of 0 to 10. She is now asking for "anything" to take away her pain and you decide that the most appropriate treatment is IV morphine. The best starting dose for Mrs. Windsor would be:

☐ a. 15 mg/hr by continuous infusion with a bolus dose of 4 mg q 15 minutes PRN.

☐ b. 12.5 mg/hr by continuous infusion with a bolus dose of 3 mg q 15 minutes PRN.

☐ c. 10 mg/hr by continuous infusion with a bolus dose of 2 mg q 15 minutes PRN.

☐ d. 24 mg/hr by continuous infusion with a bolus dose of 4 mg q 15 minutes PRN.

☐ e. 5 mg/hr by continuous infusion with a bolus dose of 1 mg q 15 minutes PRN.

(continued on next page)

Example 2-7 (continued). Medical Competence Exam for Hospice Physicians

Answer to Hospice Medical Competency Examination

Task: To convert *oral morphine* dose to *IV morphine*.

Problem: Mrs. Windsor is a 60-year-old patient with intractable pain from metastatic bone disease. She is currently using 210 mg. of MS Contin q 12 hours routinely with 60 mg MSIR ordered q 4 hours PRN for breakthrough pain. She has used 8 doses of MSIR in the past 24 hours. Despite her current medication regimen she describes her pain as constant and rates it at an "8" on a scale of 0 to 10. She is now asking for "anything" to take away her pain and you decide that the most appropriate treatment is IV morphine. The best starting dose for Mrs. Windsor would be:

☒ a. **15 mg/hr by continuous infusion with a bolus dose of 4 mg q 15 minutes PRN.**

☐ b. 12.5 mg/hr by continuous infusion with a bolus dose of 3 mg q 15 minutes PRN.

☐ c. 10 mg/hr by continuous infusion with a bolus dose of 2 mg q 15 minutes PRN.

☐ d. 24 mg/hr by continuous infusion with a bolus dose of 4 mg q 15 minutes PRN.

☐ e. 5 mg/hr by continuous infusion with a bolus dose of 1 mg q 15 minutes PRN.

The best answer is *choice A* in the above example even though it would still represent a very slight underdosing for Mrs. Windsor.

Calculations:

210 mg $\times$ 2 = 420 mg MS Contin per day

60 mg $\times$ 8 = 480 mg MSIR per day

420 + 480 = 900 mg morphine per day

Total dose of Oral Morphine per day = 900 mg

900 mg $\div$ 3 = **300 mg which represents the Oral to IV equivalency**

300 mg $\div$ 24 hours = **12.5 mg. is the hourly IV infusion rate** which would be the *equivalent* of the oral morphine dose that Mrs. Windsor was receiving. This dose has been inadequate for pain control and a *20–25%* increase in pain medication would be appropriate for this patient.

12.5 $\times$ 25% = 3

12.5 + 3 = **15.5 mg/hr would represent the increased continuous infusion rate**

A PRN bolus dose of *approximately* ⅓ of the hourly rate should be provided.

⅓ of 15 mg = **5 mg bolus dose**

The best answer of the choices above would provide a **15mg/hr infusion rate** (a 25% increase in morphine dose) with about ⅓ of the hourly rate provided as a **4 mg PRN bolus dose**.

Source: Liz Powell, Vice President Hospice. Visiting Nurses Association of Western Pennsylvania, Butler, Pennsylvania.

Example 2-8. Direct Patient Care Competencies Broken Down by Performance Criteria

The following forms illustrate how individual competencies for a variety of patient care activities (wound care, patient transfers, IV administration with a Verifuse pump, continuous ultrasound) can be evaluated as a series of steps. Each form includes a competency statement, suggestions on how the staff member may learn the competency, and the methods that should be used for evaluation.

Wound Competency

Competency Statement: Performs wound care in the home with appropriate safety and infection control measures

Learning Option(s): Demonstration, videos, and inservices

Method(s) of Evaluation: Demonstration, formal and/or informal observation, inservice attendance record

Performance Criteria	Date Met	Employee Initials	Qualified Observer Initials
Hands washed before and after client contact			
Wound care procedure reviewed			
Equipment/supplies assembled on clean/sterile surface			
Gloves worn and changed as appropriate during procedure			
Irrigation/cleaning solutions marked with date and initials			
Medical waste properly bagged/disposed of			
Personal protective equipment used when appropriate			
Supplies stored in designated/clean area			
Supplies checked for expiration dates			
Wound size (length, width, depth) and appearance documented per protocol			

Comments:

____

____

____

Validation:

_______________________________ has competently performed each of the criteria on this checklist.
(Please print)

_______________________________   _______________________________
Employee Signature   Date   Qualified Oberver Signature   Date

(continued on next page)

Example 2-8 (continued). Direct Patient Care Competencies Broken Down by Performance Criteria

Transfers

Competency Statement: Manages safe transfers of patients

Learning Option(s): Training sessions with educator

Method(s) of Evaluation: Observation of simulated or actual transfers by qualified observer

Performance Criteria	Date Met	Employee Initials	Qualified Observer Initials
Technique for Moving Patient to Edge of Bed:			
1. Moves patient's head and shoulders toward edge of bed			
2. Moves feet and legs to edge of bed			
3. Places both arms under patient's hips			
4. Moves patient toward edge of bed			
Technique for Sitting Patient on Edge of Bed:			
1. Places one hand under the patient's shoulders			
2. Instructs patient to push elbow into bed while employee lifts shoulders with one arm and swings patient legs over edge of bed			
Technique for Assisting the Patient to Transfer From Bed to Chair:			
1. Places a chair parallel to bed as close as possible and assures chair is in locked position			
2. Places patient's feet under him			
3. Faces patient and grasps each side of rib cage			
4. Pushes knee against one of patient's knees			
5. Rocks patient forward as he comes to standing position			
6. Ensures patient knees are "locked" (full extension) while patient is standing			
7. Gives patient time to balance self			
8. Pivots patient to chair			
9. Asks patient to back up to chair and place legs against the seat			
10. Assists patient to sitting position			
Technique for Transfer by Sliding Board:			
1. Places one side of sliding board under patient's buttocks and the other side on the surface of the chair, bed, toilet, etc. to which transfer is being made			
2. Instructs patient to push up with his hands to shift his buttocks and to slide across the board to the other surface			
3. Stabilizes patient during transfer if appropriate			

(continued on next page)

Example 2-8 (continued). Direct Patient Care Competencies Broken Down by Performance Criteria

Transfers

Performance Criteria	Date Met	Employee Initials	Qualified Observer Initials

Comments:

____

____

____

Validation:

__________________________________ has competently performed each of the criteria on this checklist.
(Please print)

____   ____
Employee Signature   Date   Qualified Oberver Signature   Date

(continued on next page)

Example 2-8 (continued). Direct Patient Care Competencies Broken Down by Performance Criteria

Verifuse Pump Competency

Competency Statement: Manages nursing care in the home for patients who require IV administration with the Verifuse pump.

Learning Option(s): Training sessions with the pump. Manufacturer's guide for nursing staff. The Verifuse Operator's Manual.

Method(s) of Evaluation: Observation of simulated pump programming.

Performance Criteria	Date Met	Employee Initials	Qualified Observer Initials
1. Inserts two nine-volt batteries into the Verifuse pump while holding the stop/start button. Identifies the green flashing light as an indicator that power is supplied by the nine-volt batteries.			
2. Correctly compares programmed infusion with physician orders. Press verify button when PUMP NOW LOCKED appears. (A locked bar code does not have to be scanned with each new infusion.)			
3. Programs the pump by scanning the bar code. Verifies bar code with physician orders. Bar code must be laid on a flat surface. Press the start button when shown on display screen. Scan the bar code when shown on display screen. The red scanning light illuminates; you have 30 seconds to scan the code.			
4. Compares pump infusion parameters with the bar code.			
5. Loads and primes the administration set. Removes air from solution container prior to loading the administration set. Closes tubing clamps and spikes bag. Properly inserts cartridge securely into pump. Assures tubing is secured into the air-in-line detector. Opens the clamps and presses PRIME/BOLUS button once. Checks tubing and filter to assure all air is cleared from tubing.			
6. Starts infusion by pushing START button.			
7. Connects to the rechargeable battery pack. Identifies the steady green light as indication that the battery pack is working. Verifies that there are two battery packs in the home.			
8. Connects battery pack to battery charger and plugs in to a wall outlet.			
9. Demonstrates changing/clearing a locked infusion protocol. (You have only 4 seconds to scan the bar code.)			
10. Verbalizes understanding of pump alarms (refers to Verifuse guide).			

(continued on next page)

Example 2-8 (continued). Direct Patient Care Competencies Broken Down by Performance Criteria

Verifuse Pump Competency

Performance Criteria	Date Met	Employee Initials	Qualified Observer Initials

Comments:

____

____

____

Validation:

______________________________________ has competently performed each of the criteria on this checklist.
(Please print)

_______________________________________   _______________________________________
Employee Signature   Date   Qualified Oberver Signature   Date

(continued on next page)

Example 2-8 (continued). Direct Patient Care Competencies Broken Down by Performance Criteria

Continuous Ultrasound

Competency Statement: Demonstrates proper technique in operation of continuous ultrasound

Learning Option(s): Demonstration by qualified therapist

Method(s) of Evaluation: Demonstration, formal and/or informal observation

Performance Criteria	Date Met	Employee Initials	Qualified Observer Initials
Prior to treatment checks unit to be used: Unit is grounded, face of transducer is clean, switches in off position, transducer and plug connections are tight.			
Checks that all necessary material is ready to use, such as coupling medium, towel, electrode, etc. (A commercially made gel is the preferred coupling medium, lotion may be used, mineral oil is least desirable.)			
Explains procedure to client (length of procedure, whether client will experience sensation, instructs client to tell therapist immediately if pain is experienced).			
Assesses area to be treated: • skin is clean and dry • assesses skin sensation (verbalizes that if client has poor sensation, to use low intensity setting) • verbalizes to avoid treating over abrasions or recent scar tissue • verbalizes to avoid treating over bony prominence			
Verbalizes never to treat any part of client who has an external or implanted pacemaker (superficial heat should be used).			
Instructs client that therapist will place gel on his skin. Applies gel to area to be treated.			
Turns on unit.			
Sets unit automatic timer to desired treatment time, takes into account that treatments are usually 5–8 minutes, depending upon area to be covered.			
Instructs client that transducer will feel cold. (Therapist can hold face of transducer in palm of hand for 30 seconds to warm it.)			
Applies a firm but not heavy pressure of transducer to skin.			
Verbalizes that lack of sufficient contact with coupling medium can cause periosteal pain.			
Adjusts intensity control to the desired watts per square centimeter (usually 1–2 w/cm^2) with transducer constantly moving and in firm contact with the skin.			

(continued on next page)

Example 2-8 (continued). Direct Patient Care Competencies Broken Down by Performance Criteria

Continuous Ultrasound

Performance Criteria	Date Met	Employee Initials	Qualified Observer Initials
Moves transducer in either small circular movements or small longitudinal strokes. (Speed of stroke is slow.)			
Demonstrates termination of treatment: • verbalizes that the unit will shut off automatically at completion of the treatment time • turns off intensity control • wipes off coupling medium from the transducer and replaces it in its holder • turns off unit, unplugs cord and moves unit away from the client • wipes off coupling medium from the skin (verbalizes to use alcohol if mineral oil has been used) • checks client's skin for any changes in color or texture (reddening, blisters, etc.) which is different than initial assessment			
Verbalizes that ultrasound should not be used in the following areas: • near the heart • over the eyes • on the head • near external reproductive organs • over implants • over growing bones in children • where skin suffers from any sensory impairment • over areas of malignancies • in the area of visceral plexus and large autonomous ganglion			
Verbalizes that excessive doses of ultrasound can cause damage to tissue. Periosteal pain is an indication of excess intensity and if it occurs, the power should be reduced or the application should be moved faster over the area to be treated or changed to pulse ultrasound.			
Verbalizes process of cleaning equipment between patients and upon return to supply room. (70% alcohol or disinfectant spray is to be used before replacing equipment in supply area or taking to another client.)			
Verbalizes that checklist is in the supply room and that it must be marked when equipment leaves the office and when equipment is cleaned.			
Verbalizes appropriate process for reporting defective equipment.			

(continued on next page)

Example 2-8 (continued). Direct Patient Care Competencies Broken Down by Performance Criteria

Continuous Ultrasound

Performance Criteria	Date Met	Employee Initials	Qualified Observer Initials

Comments:

____

____

____

Validation:

_________________________________ has competently performed each of the criteria on this checklist.
    (Please print)

____   ____
Employee Signature   Date   Qualified Oberver Signature   Date

Source: Home Health Services of Williamsburg Community Hospital, Williamsburg, VA.

Section 3: Maintaining and Improving Staff Competence

Examples in this section pertain to the collection, aggregation, analysis, and trending of competence data to identify ongoing education and training needs. Some methods for record keeping can be useful both in data collection and in demonstrating compliance with Joint Commission standards dealing with competence assessment.

Example 3-1. Self-Assessment Form for Gathering Data

This self-assessment checklist can be given to new employees during orientation or to current staff during competence assessment to gather data on areas in which staff might need individualized training or ongoing education. Although the form primarily covers technical skills, it could be expanded to include other areas such as developing a plan of care, completing a Medicare 485 form or certificate of medical necessity, and developing drug monographs or pharmacokinetic monitoring parameters. This form is only useful if the data gathered are aggregated, analyzed, and trended for review and use by leaders in planning and improving the competence assessment program.

RN Competency Checklist

Name ____   Title ________________________

PROCEDURE	Exp.	Need Exp.	No Experience
Mechanical Equipment			
Infusion Pumps			
Enteral Pump (Kangaroo)			
Doppler Monitors (Fetal)			
Pulse Oximeter			
Blood Glucose Monitor			
Infusion Therapy			
Peripheral — Insertion, Maintenance, Discontinuation			
Central Line — Management			
care & use of Hickman			
care & use of Groshong			
care & use of Triple Lumen Catheter			
care & use of Infusion Ports			
Heparin Lock			
medication administration			
maintenance			
Teaching Client/Caregiver			
Naso-Gastric Tube Feeding			
Placement of NG tube			
Gastric Lavage			
Gastric Gavage			

(continued on next page)

Example 3-1 (continued). Self-Assessment Form for Gathering Data

RN Competency Checklist

PROCEDURE	Exp.	Need Exp.	No Experience
Naso-Gastric Tube Feeding (cont.)			
Small Bore Feeding Tube			
placement			
maintenance/removal			
Med Administration Via NG Tube			
PEG			
feeding & site care			
Nasogastric Tube			
irrigation			
Teaching Care to Client/Caregiver			
Ostomy Care			
Respiratory			
Tracheostomy			
care			
changing of tube, cuffed & non-cuffed			
Suctioning			
naso-trach suctioning			
tracheostomy & endotracheal suctioning			
O_2 Administration			
cannula, catheter			
CPAP			
nebulizers (handheld)			
O_2 Concentrators			
Transtracheal O_2			
Surgical Sites/Wounds			
Dressing Change			
sterile			
aseptic			
Removal of:			
staples			
sutures			
Wound Irrigation			
Wound Packing			
Teaching Care to Client/Caregiver			

(continued on next page)

Example 3-1 (continued). Self-Assessment Form for Gathering Data

RN Competency Checklist

PROCEDURE	Exp.	Need Exp.	No Experience
Urinary			
Suprapubic			
care, maintenance			
reinsertion			
Catheterization			
Catheter Care			
irrigation			
medication installation			
teaching self cath.			
Medication Administration			
Injections			
SQ			
IM			
z-track			
intradermal			
IV Push			
compatible sol.			
incompatible sol.			
IV Piggyback			
Oral			
Other			
eye drops & ointment			
sublingual/buccal			
transdermal patches			
rectal			
pain management			
Basic Procedures			
Universal Precautions			
AIDS			
Hep B			
home hazardous waste disposal			

Phlebotomy/Bloodwork

CPR Certification

Yes _______ No _______ Date Expires _______________________

(continued on next page)

Example 3-1 (continued). Self-Assessment Form for Gathering Data

Home Health Aide Competency Checklist

Name____   Title______________________________

PROCEDURE	Exp.	Need Exp.	No Experience
Blood Pressures			
Pulse			
Apical			
Radial			
Temp			
Oral			
Rectal			
Axillary			
Bed Bath			
Shower			
Make Occupied Bed			
ROM Exercises			
Active			
Passive			
Colostomy Care			
G-tube Care			
Foley Care			
Moving Patients			
Turning			
Dangling			
Up in Chair			
Feeding the Patient			
Assisting and Setting up Food Tray			
Feeding			
Recording Intake/Output			
Application of Elastic Stockings			
Administration of Fleets Enema			
Collection of Specimens - Urine			
Routine			
Clean Catch			
Testing Specimens - Urine			
Clintest & Acetest (C & A)			
Basic Procedures - Universal Precautions			
AIDS			
Hep B			
Hazardous Waste Disposal			

CPR Certification

Yes _______   No _______   Date Expires ______________________________

Example 3-2. HME Staff Education and Competence Records

The policy, guidelines, and form shown here are helpful for keeping records of individual staff competence assessments and ongoing education in a central, easily accessed location. Keeping these records up to date makes it easier to aggregate data for leaders to review during planning activities. The information is also readily available when it is time for the organization's accreditation survey.

Title: Education Competency Records

Home Care
Home Medical Equipment
Page 1 of 1
Effective Date: _________________
Approved By: _________________

I. Policy:

A complete and current record of all continuing education programs attended and competencies achieved by team members shall be maintained and available for review by appropriate regulatory agencies.

II. Purpose

To ensure knowledge and skill necessary to perform job responsibilities.

III. Guidelines:

1. An Education/Competency Record for each team member for the current year shall be maintained in the Education Binder in the "Off Stage" area.

2. Each team member is responsible to keep his/her Education/Competency Record current.

3. Competency checks are to be performed based on the skills required for the position.

4. During the team member's performance appraisal, the manager will verify with the team member that his/her record is up to date.

5. Education records for the current year are kept in the department. Records from previous years are sent to the Personnel Department for filing in the master personnel files.

(continued on next page)

Example 3-2 (continued). HME Staff Education and Competence Records

Home Care
Home Medical Equipment
Education/Competency Record
1994

Name: ____   Position: _______________________________

Attended Act I & II: ______________________________________   Date Employed: _______________________

Mandatory Programs/Inservices	Date	Verified
Infection Control — Department Specific		
Fire Safety — Hospital Wide		
Fire Safety — Department Specific		
Electrical Safety — Hospital Wide		
Electrical Safety — Department Specific		
M.S.D.S. — Hospital Wide		
M.S.D.S. — Department Specific		
Back Safety — Hospital Wide		
Back Safety — Department Specific		
Confidentiality		
Emergency Preparedness		
Severe Weather		
Rights & Responsibilities		

Committees: ____

____

____

Professional Organization Memberships: ____

____

____

____

Certifications:

____   Exp. Date _______________________

____   Exp. Date _______________________

(continued on next page)

Example 3-2 (continued). HME Staff Education and Competence Records

Home Care
Home Medical Equipment
Education/Competency Record
1994

Competencies	Date	Verified
Oxygen Analyzer		
Cylinder Oxygen		
Liquid Oxygen Transfill		
Liquid Oxygen Set-up		
Oxygen Concentrator Set-up		
C.P.A.P. Set-up		
Apnea Monitor Set-up		

Inservices Attended	Date

Source: Margaret Scallan, RN, Administrative Director, East Jefferson General Hospital, Home Care Network, Metairie, Louisiana.

Example 3-3. **Educational Materials for Staff Caring for Age-Specific Populations**

Four age-specific learning modules are used by this organization to orient and train staff in care practices for these specific populations. In addition to the modules for infancy and adolescence, shown here, materials cover childhood and adult patients. Each module defines the age parameters of the group; motor, cognitive, psychosocial, physical, and other characteristics; and a post-test to evaluate staff's understanding of the material.

Age Specific Learning Module
Infancy (Birth–12 Months)

Motor	Cognitive	Psychosocial	Physical	Other
Birth–1 Month • Visually fixes on objects and faces. • Lies on back with head averted. • Keeps hands fisted. **1–3 Months** • Hands begin to come to face. • Will take objects and move them to mouth. • Begins to hold head up when placed prone. • Turns from side to back. • Eyes follow better and will focus.	**Birth–1 Month** • Responses limited to tension states and discomfort. • Likes feeding, bathing, cuddling, and being rocked. • Quiets when picked up. **1–3 Months** • Recognizes familiar faces. • More aware and interested in environment. • Enjoys sucking— puts hands in mouth.	**Birth–1 Month** • Cries and makes discriminating sounds. • Sleeps long intervals. **1–3 Months** • Begins vocalization, babbles and coos. • Begins social smile. • Crying becomes differentiated. • Eyes may follow person or object more intently. • May become aware of new situations. • Gets pleasure from sucking, putting hands in mouth. • May start to establish sleep routine.	**Birth–1 Month** • Eyes follow objects. • Requires more fluid relative to size than adults. • Feeding schedule according to infant needs. May have breast milk or formula followed by water. **1–3 Months** • Anticipates and enjoys feedings. • Posterior fontanelle closes at about 3 months. Anterior fontanelle remains open. • Average weekly weight gain 4–7 ounces. • Average height gain 1 inch per month.	In infancy, severe illnesses may produce intense emotional reactions in new parents at the very time they are trying to become a family, rather than a marital couple. Parents with little child-rearing experience have great difficulty separating problems with their baby into illness-related and normal disturbances. In some cases, the predictable guilt, horror, and disbelief associated with illness or handicap in an infant can damage parental-child attachment, leading to chronic dysfunction. Generally, ultimate adaption is good, and some follow-up studies of oncology survivors have found that the earlier the illness, the better the long-term functioning (Koocher, et al. 1980). **Normal Ranges for Vital Signs, Height, and Weight** ***Temperatures (Rectal)*** Newborn 97.7–98.6F 3 months 99.4F 6 months 99.3F 1 year 99.7F ***Respiratory Rate*** 30–60 Breaths Per Minute

(continued on next page)

Example 3-3 (continued). Educational Materials for Staff Caring for Age-Specific Populations

Age Specific Learning Module
Infancy (Birth–12 Months)

Motor	Cognitive	Psychosocial	Physical	Other
4–7 Months • Eyes focus on small objects. • Holds head up when pulled to sitting position. • Hands may come to meet rattle, grasping with both hands. • Sits with minimal support. • Begins to roll over. • May begin crawling or scooting. **8–12 Months** • Sits without support, recovers balance. • Manipulates objects with hands. • Pulls self up in crib. • Does not like supine position. • May be crawling, walking, and climbing. • May begin throwing objects.	**4–7 Months** • Interested in environment. • Recognizes bottle. • Becomes bored, enjoys attention. • May sleep through night. • Searches for lost objects, drops and picks up objects. • Exhibits some fear of strangers. **8–12 Months** • Responds to own name. • Points to indicate wants. • Has increased attention span. • Begins to imitate.	**4–7 Months** • Laughs and chuckles. • Fussing for a reason. • May say recognizable words, makes talking sounds in response to others. • Discriminates between familiar faces and strangers. • May respond to "no-no". • Enjoys being propped in sitting position, likes highchair. **8–12 Months** • Smiles at images in mirror. • Strong urge toward independence in dressing, eating, and moving. • Shows fear, anger, affection, jealousy, anxiety, and sympathy.	**4–7 Months** • May start teething. • Begins eating cereal and strained fruits in addition to formula or breast milk. • May start drinking from a cup. • Weight and height gains continue. **8–12 Months** • Holds bottle and may feed self crackers. • May use spoon and cup. • Eating mashed table foods or junior foods. Likes finger foods. • Usually begins drinking cow's milk. • May have regular bowel movements. • Continues teething.	**Normal Ranges for Vital Signs, Height, and Weight (continued)** *Heart Rate* *Awake* *Sleeping* Neonate 100–180 80–160 Infant 100–160 75–160 *Blood Pressures* 0–1 month 76/68–98/65 1–3 months 100/64 4–7 months 106/66 8–12 months 106/66 *Weights (kg)* 0–1 month 4 kg 1–3 months 4–5 kg 4–7 months 5–8 kg 8–12 months 9–11 kg *Heights (cms)* *Girls* 0–1 month 54–56 cms 1–3 months 56–68 cms 4–7 months 61–68 cms 8–12 months 70–77 cms *Boys* 0–1 month 51–59 cms 1–3 months 59–66 cms 4–7 months 68–73 cms 8–12 months 74–80 cms

(continued on next page)

Example 3-3 (continued). Educational Materials for Staff Caring for Age-Specific Populations

Age Specific Learning Module
Infancy (Birth–12 Months)

Motor	Cognitive	Psychosocial	Physical	Other
				Normal Ranges for Vital Signs, Height, and Weight (continued) ***Usual Sequence of Tooth Eruption (Primary Dentition)*** *Maxillary* 1. Central Incisor — 8–12 months 2. Lateral Incisor — 10–12 months 3. Cuspid — 18–24 months 4. First molar — 12–15 months 5. Second molar — 24–30 months *Mandibular* 6. Central Incisor — 5–9 months 7. Lateral Incisor — 12–15 months 8. Cuspid — 18–24 months 9. First molar — 12–15 months 10. Second molar — 24–30 months

(continued on next page)

Example 3-3 (continued). Educational Materials for Staff Caring for Age-Specific Populations

Age Specific Learning Module
Infancy (Birth–12 Months)

Motor	Cognitive	Psychosocial	Physical	Other
				Recognizing Child Abuse Parent, child, and environment—all generally contribute to child abuse situations. The checklists below detail some observable characteristics of abusive parents and abused children. Of course, the presence of any of these factors doesn't automatically indicate child abuse, but it does suggest that you should investigate further. Because child abuse occurs more frequently in high-crime areas and crowded urban communities, many people associate it only with poorly educated, socio-economically disadvantaged families. Don't be blinded by this stereotype—it's increasingly yielding to evidence that child abuse also occurs in middle and upper income families, among seemingly well adjusted parents and children. Characteristics the abusive parent may exhibit: • Lacks knowledge of infant developmental skills. • Has unrealistic expectations of the child's behavior. • Feels intensely anxious about the child's behavior. • Feels guilty and angry about inability to provide for the child. • Feels extremely lonely and isolated.

(continued on next page)

Example 3-3 (continued). Educational Materials for Staff Caring for Age-Specific Populations

Age Specific Learning Module
Infancy (Birth–12 Months)

Motor	Cognitive	Psychosocial	Physical	Other
				Recognizing Child Abuse (continued) • Relates poorly with spouse and own parents. • Has also been a victim of child abuse. • Believes physical punishment is the best discipline. • Lacks a strong emotional attachment to the child (for example, a mother who hasn't bonded well with her child). Characteristics the abused child may exhibit: • Has a history of behavior problems. • Is overactive, demanding, defiant. • Refuses to eat, violates rules, destroys parent's property and the property of others.

References Used for Age Specific Learning Modules

Brunner LS, Smith D: *The Lippincott Manual of Nursing Practice*, Philadelphia: JB Lippincott Company, 1991.

Chenitz WC, Stone JT, Salisbury SA: *Clinical Gerontological Nursing*. Philadelphia: WB Saunders, 1991.

Erickson E: *Childhood and Society*. London: Penguin Co, 1965.

Greene MG: *The Harriet Lane Handbook*. St. Louis: Mosby-Year Book, 1991.

Hay W, et al: *Current Pediatrics Diagnosis and Treatment*. Stanford, CT: Appleton & Lang, 1995.

Jarvis C: *Physical Examination and Health Assessment*. Philadelphia: WB Saunders, 1995.

Kriston JM: Contemporary Ericksonian Theory: A psychobiographical illustration. *Gerontology and Geriatrics Education* 14(4): 81–91, 1994.

Weiner JM: *Textbook of Childhood and Adolescent Psychiatry*. Washington, DC: American Psychiatric Press, 1993.

White L: *Growth and Development in Basic Nursing Skills and Concepts*, St. Louis: Mosby-Year Book, 1991.

(continued on next page)

Example 3-3 (continued). Educational Materials for Staff Caring for Age-Specific Populations

Name: _______________________________

Social Security #: _______________________

Unit: _______________________________

Date: _______________________________

Post-Test
Infancy
(Birth to 12 Months)

Circle the correct answer.

1. Children 8–12 months eat mashed table foods or junior foods.

    T   F

2. An infant 1–3 months anticipates and enjoys feedings.

    T   F

3. Parents with little child-rearing experience have great difficulty separating problems with their baby into illness-related and normal disturbances.

    T   F

4. An infant under 1 month of age requires more fluid relative to size than adults.

    T   F

(continued on next page)

Example 3-3 (continued). Educational Materials for Staff Caring for Age-Specific Populations

Age Specific Learning Module
Adolescence (13 Years–15 Years)

Motor	Cognitive	Psychosocial	Physical	Other
• Muscular ability and coordination increase. • Energy is increased as growth spurt ends.	• Begins abstract and analytical thinking. • Thoughtful—needs to be included in making decisions about care.	• Increased interest in opposite sex. • Sensitive about body issues. • Needs privacy protected. • Peer group more important than family. • Changing from dependent to independent. • May relieve tension by "goofing off." • Takes risks/seeks thrills. • Values truth and justice. Wants honesty from caregivers.	• Phase of development begins when reproductive organs become functionally operative; phase ends when physical growth is completed. • Hands and feet growing. • Large muscles develop, begin increased coordination.	**Teens** In teenagers, illnesses can impact on their struggle for autonomy, their physical-sexuality development, and their peer relationships. Illness can force dependance on parents and physicians to a degree not found in healthy teenagers. The perception of immaturity by adults, due to delayed growth in secondary sexual characteristics, can reinforce this dependence. Compliance problems often result when the illness and its treatment become involved in a teenager's conflictual struggle for independence. Fully developed autonomy actually enhances the teenager's adoption of reasonable therapeutic goals. Likewise, compliance with salicylate therapy in teenagers with rheumatoid arthritis increases with better developed autonomy (Litt, et al. 1982). Physical and sexual maturation may be delayed by chronic illness. Boys who are late in developing are rated as less mature, popular, or confident than their peers. For girls, maturing at the same rate as their peers is associated with greatest confidence (Gross and Duke 1980). Family reactions to an ill child are equally complex and dependent on prior family patterns, coping styles, and experiences with illness. Reactions of fear, anger, loneliness, and guilt seem universal (Featherstone 1980).

(continued on next page)

Example 3-3 (continued). Educational Materials for Staff Caring for Age-Specific Populations

Age Specific Learning Module
Adolescence (13 Years–15 Years)

Motor	Cognitive	Psychosocial	Physical	Other
				Teens (continued) Marital strain seems inevitable, and some research (Breslau and Davis 1986) has found a grater rate of divorce and depressive symptoms in mothers of children with chronic illness. For many illnesses, such as cancer and AIDS, the ambiguity and social anxiety are unsettling (Comaroff and Maguire 1981; Krener and Miller 1989). In the face of acute illness, siblings can be relatively neglected by parents and health care workers. Reactions of jealousy, overprotectiveness, and survival guilt are common. Some programs for the chronically ill have specific components for siblings to address these issues. **Normal Ranges for Vital Signs, Height, and Weight** *Blood Pressures* Girls　124/78–126/82 Boys　124/77–129/79 *Height (feet)* Girls　4½–5 feet Boys　4½–5 feet 9 inches *Weight (lbs)* Girls　139–154 lbs Boys　136–163 lbs

(continued on next page)

Example 3-3 (continued). Educational Materials for Staff Caring for Age-Specific Populations

Age Specific Learning Module
Adolescence (13 Years–15 Years)

Motor	Cognitive	Psychosocial	Physical	Other
				Normal Ranges for Vital Signs, Height, and Weight (continued) ***Pulse*** *(13–15 years)* Girls 70–110 Boys 65–105 *(16 years)* Girls 60–100 Boys 55–95 ***Respiratory Rate*** 18–20 Caregivers should have a "high index" of suspicion for drug abuse among all adolescents but particularly among the following: • Children of substance abusers • Victims of physical, sexual, or psycho-social abuse • School dropouts • Pregnant teenagers • Economically disadvantaged youth • Antisocial and delinquent youth • Youth with mental health problems (especially depressed and suicidal youth) • Physically disabled youth

(continued on next page)

Example 3-3 (continued). Educational Materials for Staff Caring for Age-Specific Populations

Name: _______________________________

Social Security #: _______________________________

Unit: _______________________________

Date: _______________________________

Post-Test
Adolescence
(13 Years–15 Years)

Circle the correct answer.

1. The 13–15 year old expects caregivers to provide information with truth and honesty.

    T   F

2. Adolescents should be provided privacy because of sensitivity about their bodies.

    T   F

3. In teenagers, illnesses can impact on their struggle for autonomy, their physical and sexual development, and their peer relationships.

    T   F

4. The 13–15 year old adolescents do which of the following?

    a. Are interested in the opposite sex.

    b. Prefer family over peer group.

    c. Remain dependent on family.

    d. Still think concretely.

Source: Floanne Hinton Micks, Director, Staff Development, Riverside Regional Medical Center, Newport News, VA.

Example 3-4. **Aggregation of Annual Competence Evaluations**

This form, which can be expanded and adapted for any type of service, shows one way to collect data on organizationwide staff competence. Each of the main areas (infection control, assessment of home environment, patient education, equipment management, and clinical procedures) can be broken down into more specific components as needed. By recording the total number of employees assessed for each of these competencies and the number who showed a need for improvement, leaders can see where resources for additional training and education need to be allocated.

Annual Competency Report Form

Date: _____________   Completed by: _____________

	Assessment	Clinical Procedures	Equipment Management	Infection Control	Patient Education
Total number of employees assessed					
Number of employees showing need for improvement					
Areas most commonly cited as opportunities for improvement					
Most important area to be addressed in training and inservices					

APPENDIX

Fulfilling the items on this list should help readers ensure they are prepared to demonstrate compliance with the Joint Commission's home care competency standards.

______ Have we identified the competence-related components in the management of human resources standards in the *Comprehensive Accreditation Manual for Home Care*?

______ Have we studied the standards, intents, and other materials to ensure we understand the requirements?

______ Have we performed a self-assessment to determine compliance with the competency standards? Did the self-assessment cover

      ______ planning for competent staff

      ______ assessing competence for all patient care staff

      ______ staff development programs aimed at maintaining and improving competence?

______ Have we identified the documents required for the document and record review activities?

______ Have we assigned responsibility within our organization for collecting the documents required for the document and record review activities, including records related to contracted staff?

______ Have we labeled each document for the document review session according to the standard it fulfills?

______ Have we identified the individuals from our organization who will participate in each competence-related survey activity?

      ______ Leadership interviews

      ______ Clinical supervisor interviews

      ______ Patient care staff interviews

      ______ Document review

      ______ Personnel record review

      ______ Home visits

______ Have we discussed and rehearsed the key points we would like to communicate to surveyors during each of these activities?

      ______ Leadership interviews

      ______ Clinical supervisor interviews

      ______ Patient care staff interviews

      ______ Document review

      ______ Personnel record review

      ______ Home visits

______ Have we prepared patient care staff for surveyor participation in home visits?

Annotated Bibliography

Benefield LE: Productivity in home healthcare: Assessing nurse effectiveness and efficiency. Part One. *Home Healthc Nurse* 14(9):698–706, 1996.

Describes the development of a profile of the specific knowledge, skills, and abilities (competencies) exhibited by "productive" registered nurses and illustrates how this profile can be used as a basis for developing the home health nurse's job description, hiring and interviewing guidelines, and performance appraisal forms. The tables showing the proficiencies that make up the Productivity Measurement Classification provide excellent examples of different areas to consider in competency assessment.

Broadwell MM: Seven steps to building better training. *Training* 30:75–81, Oct 1993.

Outlines a seven-step process for establishing an effective training program, including specific questions that may be asked and required actions.

Byrum CD, Rudisill PT, Singletary MB: The traveling salvation show: A performance-centered skills fair. *J Nurs Staff Dev* 12: 198–203, 1996.

The traveling salvation show is an innovative approach to reviewing high-risk/low-frequency skills for nurses on critical care units. Although it focuses on an acute care setting, the description of the program, how it was developed, how it is used to meet Joint Commission competency standards, and the successful outcomes it has achieved provide helpful examples that can be adapted and applied to many types of home care organizations. The focus on critical thinking and performance-centered learning are especially noteworthy.

del Bueno DJ, Griffin LR, Burke SM, Foley MA: The clinical teacher: A critical link in competence development. *J Nurs Staff Dev* 6:135–138, 1990.

This article describes the need for collaboration between an organization's education and clinical staff to ensure that knowledge translates effectively into high-quality performance of care and services. The report focuses on one method that was found effective—Performance-Based Development Systems (PBDS).

Friedman MM: Competence assessment: How to meet the intent of the Joint Commission on Accreditation of Healthcare Organization's Management of Human Resources standards. *Home Healthc Nurse* 14(10):771–774, 1996.

Summarizes the requirements of the competency assessment standards and the basic steps to meet these requirements. Good general information based on the 1995 home care standards.

Garland GA: Self report of competence: A tool for the staff development specialist. *J Nurs Staff Dev* 12: 191–197, 1996.

Specifically geared for those involved in staff training and education, this article reports on a study of nurses' self-assessment data being used in the development of competency-based education programs. Findings and suggestions, although based on medical-surgical nurse responses, may provide ideas for using similar tools as part of the data collection, analysis, and trending necessary to identify other staff's learning needs.

Johnson ME: Performance architecture for home care agencies. *CARING* 15: 54–57, May 1996.

Explains a strategy for improving staff capabilities in order to improve the overall efficiency and competitiveness of a home care agency (performance architecture) and illustrates the relationship between performance improvement and competency. Defines performance management (the work staff members perform) and professional development (how competent that performance is) as the basis of performance architecture and describes steps an organization may take in creating an effective system of assessing, maintaining, and improving competencies based on its goals and standards.

Robinson SM and Barberis-Ryan C: Competency assessment: A systematic approach. *Nurs Manage* 26(2):40–44.

Describes how one organization adapted an existing clinical development plan as a framework for its own competency assessment program. Levels of nurse competencies were identified, and each competency had a technical, interpersonal, and critical-thinking component. The overall process is described, and examples of implementation are provided.

Sullivan CA: Competency assessment and performance improvement for healthcare providers. *JHQ* 16(4):14–19, 38, July/Aug 1994.

Proposes a three-part model to ensure competency assessment and performance improvement are integrated in a program that addresses all types of healthcare providers. The model includes a skills inventory, a standards review to promote compliance, and a peer review program. Most of the examples pertain to physicians and nurses, but sample inventories of skills can be adapted to many categories of home care professionals.

Twardon C, Gartner M, Cherry C: A competency achievement orientation program: Professional development of the home health nurse. *JONA* 23(7/8):20–25, July/Aug 1993.

Describes the Home Nursing Agency's program to meet the needs of newly employed registered nurses, which facilitates the development of independent practice and judgment skills. Illustrates the importance of competency-based orientation programs for home health nurses.

INDEX

A

B

C

D